Structural Heart Cases

A COLOR ATLAS OF PEARLS AND PITFALLS

Structural Heart Cases

A COLOR ATLAS OF PEARLS AND PITFALLS

PAUL SORAJJA, MD
Director, Center for Valve and Structural Heart Disease
Minneapolis Heart Institute
Abbott Northwestern Hospital
Minneapolis, Minnesota

ELSEVIER

ELSEVIER

1600 John F. Kennedy Blvd.
Ste 1800
Philadelphia, PA 19103-2899

STRUCTURAL HEART CASES: A COLOR ATLAS OF PEARLS
AND PITFALLS

ISBN: 978-0-323-54695-9

Notices

Knowledge and best practice in this field are constantly changing. As new research and experience
broaden our understanding, changes in research methods, professional practices, or medical treatment may
become necessary.

Practitioners and researchers must always rely on their own experience and knowledge in evaluating
and using any information, methods, compounds, or experiments described herein. In using such
information or methods they should be mindful of their own safety and the safety of others, including
parties for whom they have a professional responsibility.

With respect to any drug or pharmaceutical products identified, readers are advised to check the most
current information provided (i) on procedures featured or (ii) by the manufacturer of each product to be
administered, to verify the recommended dose or formula, the method and duration of administration, and
contraindications. It is the responsibility of practitioners, relying on their own experience and knowledge
of their patients, to make diagnoses, to determine dosages and the best treatment for each individual
patient, and to take all appropriate safety precautions.

To the fullest extent of the law, neither the Publisher nor the authors, contributors, or editors, assume
any liability for any injury and/or damage to persons or property as a matter of products liability,
negligence or otherwise, or from any use or operation of any methods, products, instructions, or ideas
contained in the material herein.

Library of Congress Cataloging-in-Publication Data

Names: Sorajja, Paul, author.
Title: Structural heart cases : a color atlas of pearls and pitfalls / Paul Sorajja.
Description: Philadelphia, PA : Elsevier, [2019] | Includes index.
Identifiers: LCCN 2017041757 | ISBN 9780323546959 (pbk. : alk. paper)
Subjects: | MESH: Heart Diseases | Case Reports | Atlases
Classification: LCC RC682 | NLM WG 17 | DDC 616.1/2—dc23 LC record available at https://lccn.loc.gov/
    2017041757

Content Strategist: Robin Carter
Content Development Manager: Lucia Gunzel
Content Development Specialist: Joan Ryan
Book Production Manager: Jeff Patterson
Project Manager: Lisa A. P. Bushey
Designer: Brian Salisbury

Printed in China

Last digit is the print number: 9   8   7   6   5   4   3   2   1

Working together
to grow libraries in
developing countries

www.elsevier.com • www.bookaid.org

To my wonderful parents, Khoontol and Pornpimol Sorajja, who showed me what I could not see myself.

To my loving daughters, Natali and Amalin Sorajja, who represent all that is good in the world now and in the future.

And to the love of my life, Abbie Lea Young, who continues to inspire me to expand my personal boundaries and dream of expanding those of others.

List of Contributors

Samer Abbas, MD
Interventional Cardiology
Director, Cardiovascular Service
Director, Cath Lab
Community Hospital
Munster, Indiana

Shuaib Abdullah, MD, MSCs
VA North Texas Healthcare System
University of Texas Southwestern Medical Center
Dallas, Texas

Hasan Ahmad, MD
Division of Cardiology
Westchester Medical Center
Valhalla, New York

Gorav Ailawadi, MD
Chief, Division of Cardiovascular Surgery
Professor, Cardiac Surgery and Biomedical Engineering
Director, Minimally Invasive Cardiac Surgery
Surgical Director, Advanced Cardiac Valve Center
Director, Surgery Innovation Center
University of Virginia
Charlottesville, Virginia

Wail Alkashkari, MD
King Faisal Cardiac Center
King Abdulaziz Medical City for National Guard
Jeddah, Saudi Arabia

Osama Alsanjari, MD
Sussex Cardiac Centre
Brighton and Sussex University Hospitals
Brighton, United Kingdom

Jason H. Anderson, MD
Assistant Professor of Pediatrics
Senior Associate Consultant
Division of Pediatric Cardiology
Mayo Clinic
Rochester, Minnesota

Judah Askew, MD
Cardiac Surgeon
Minneapolis Heart Institute
Abbott Northwestern Hospital
Minneapolis, Minnesota

Luis Asmarats, MD
Quebec Heart and Lung Institute
Laval University
Quebec City, Quebec, Canada

Ganesh Athappan, MD
Minneapolis Heart Institute
Abbott Northwestern Hospital
Minneapolis, Minnesota

Rizwan Attia, PhD, MRCS
Department of Cardiothoracic Surgery
Barts Heart Centre
London, United Kingdom

Vasilis Babaliaros, MD
Associate Professor of Medicine
Division of Cardiology
Emory University
Atlanta, Georgia

Richard Y. Bae, MD
Director, Echocardiography Laboratory
Director, Interventional Echocardiography
Minneapolis Heart Institute at Abbott Northwestern Hospital
Minneapolis, Minnesota

Charles M. Baker, MD
Children's Hospital
Minneapolis, Minnesota

Subhash Banerjee, MD
Chief of Cardiology
VA North Texas Healthcare System
University of Texas Southwestern Medical Center
Dallas, Texas

Vinayak N. Bapat, MCh, FRCS(CTh)
Consultant, Cardiothoracic Surgeon
Cardiothoracic Surgery
St. Thomas's Hospital
London, United Kingdom

Colin M. Barker, MD
Interventional Cardiology
Houston Methodist Hospital
Houston, Texas

Itsik Ben-Dor, MD
Associate Professor of Cardiovascular
Medicine at the Georgetown University Medical Center
MedStar Washington Hospital Center
Washington, District of Columbia

Stefan Bertog, MD, PhD
Cardiovascular Center Frankfurt
Frankfurt, Germany;
Veterans Affairs Hospital
Minneapolis, Minnesota

Phillipe Blanke, MD, PhD
Department of Cardiac Imaging
St Paul's Hospital
Vancouver, British Columbia, Canada

Peter Block, MD
Division of Cardiology
Emory University School of Medicine
Atlanta, Georgia

Patrick Boehm, MD
Cardiovascular Center Frankfurt
Frankfurt, Germany

Stephen Brecker, MD
St George's Hospital
University of London
London, United Kingdom

Emmanouil S. Brilakis, MD, PhD
Minneapolis Heart Institute
Abbott Northwestern Hospital
Minneapolis, Minnesota

Marcus Burns, DNP
Minneapolis Heart Institute
Abbott Northwestern Hospital
Minneapolis, Minnesota

Christian Butter, Prof. Dr. (MD)
Heart Center Brandenburg in Bernau
Brandenburg, Germany

Allison K. Cabalka, MD
Professor of Pediatrics
Consultant, Division of Pediatric Cardiology
Mayo Clinic College of Medicine
Rochester, Minnesota

Barry Cabuay, MD
Senior Consulting Cardiologist
Division of Cardiovascular Surgery
Minneapolis Heart Institute
Minneapolis, Minnesota

Alex Campbell, MD
Senior Consulting Cardiologist
Minneapolis Heart Institute
Minneapolis, Minnesota

John D. Carroll, MD
Professor of Medicine
University of Colorado
Denver, Colorado;
Director of Interventional Cardiology
Anschutz Medical Campus
Aurora, Colorado

Anson W. Cheung, MD, BSc, MSc, FRCSC
Clinical Professor
Surgical Director, Cardiac Transplant Program of BC
St. Paul's Hospital
Vancouver, British Columbia, Canada

Adnan K. Chhatriwalla, MD
Associate Professor of Medicine
University of Missouri–Kansas City
Medical Director, Structural Intervention
Saint Luke's Mid America Heart Institute
Kansas City, Missouri

Martin Cohen, MD
Division of Cardiology
Westchester Medical Center
Valhalla, New York

Mauricio G. Cohen, MD
Associate Professor of Medicine
University of Miami Miller School of Medicine
Director, Cardiac Catheterization Laboratory
University of Miami Hospital and Clinics
Miami, Florida

Frank Corrigan, MD
Division of Cardiology
Emory University School of Medicine
Atlanta, Georgia

Cameron Dowling, MBBS
St George's Hospital
University of London
London, United Kingdom

Tanya Dutta, MD, MA
Westchester Medical Center
New York Medical College
Valhalla, New York

Mackram Eleid, MD
Associate Professor of Medicine
Department of Cardiovascular Medicine
College of Medicine
Mayo Clinic
Rochester, Minnesota

Robert Saeid Farivar, MD, PhD
Section of Cardiac Surgery
Minneapolis Heart Institute
Abbott Northwestern Hospital
Minneapolis, Minnesota

Ted Feldman, MD
Director, Cardiac Catheterization Laboratories
Evanston Hospital, Cardiology Division
Evanston, Illinois

Thomas Flavin, MD
Section of Cardiac Surgery
Minneapolis Heart Institute
Minneapolis, Minnesota

Jessica Forcillo, MD
Division Cardiothoracic Surgery
Emory University School of Medicine
Atlanta, Georgia

Jennifer Franke, MD
Cardiovascular Center Frankfurt
Frankfurt, Germany

Sameer Gafoor, MD
Medical Director, Structural Heart Disease
Cardiology
Swedish Medical Center
Seattle, Washington

Evaldas Girdauskas, MD, PhD
Surgical Director
Minimally Invasive Valve Surgery Program
Department of Cardiovascular Surgery
University Heart Center Hamburg
Hamburg, Germany

Steven L. Goldberg, MD
Director, Structural Heart Disease
Community Hospital of the Monterey Peninsula (CHOMP)
Monterey, California;
Chief Medical Officer, Cardiac Dimensions
Kirkland, Washington

Mario Gössl, MD, PhD
Director, Transcatheter Research and Education
Program Director, Structural Interventional Fellowship
Senior Consulting Cardiologist
Minneapolis Heart Institute
Abbott Northwestern Hospital
Minneapolis, Minnesota

Mayra Guerrero, MD
Director of Cardiac Structural Interventions
Evanston Hospital
Evanston, Illinois;
Clinical Associate Professor of Medicine
Pritzker School of Medicine
University of Chicago
Chicago, Illinois

Alexander Haak, PhD
Philips Healthcare
Andover, Massachusetts

Cameron Hague, MD
Department of Cardiac Imaging
St. Paul's Hospital
Vancouver, British Columbia, Canada

Eva Harmel, MD
Department of Cardiac Surgery
University Heart Center Hamburg
Hamburg, Germany

Ziyad Hijazi, MD
Professor of Pediatrics
Weill Cornell Medicine
Chair, Department of Pediatrics
Director, Sidra Cardiac Program
Editor-in-Chief, Journal of Structural Heart Disease
New York, New York;
Sidra Medical and Research Center
Doha, Qatar

David Hildick-Smith, MD, FRCP
Professor of Interventional Cardiology
Sussex Cardiac Centre
Brighton and Sussex University Hospitals
Brighton, United Kingdom

Ilona Hofmann, MD
Cardiovascular Center Frankfurt
Frankfurt, Germany

Samuel E. Horr, MD
Cleveland Clinic
Cleveland, Ohio

Nay M. Htun, MBBS, MRCP(UK), FRACP, PhD
St. Paul's Hospital
Vancouver, British Columbia, Canada

Shaw Hua (Anthony) Kueh, MBChB, FRACP
Department of Cardiology
Auckland City Hospital
Auckland, New Zealand

Vladimir Jelnin, MD
Division of Cardiology
North Shore Health System
Lenox Hill Heart and Vascular Institute of New York
New York, New York

Brandon M. Jones, MD
Fellow, Interventional Cardiology
Cardiovascular Medicine
Cleveland Clinic
Cleveland, Ohio

Ravi Joshi, MD
VA North Texas Healthcare System
University of Texas Southwestern Medical Center
Dallas, Texas

Rami Kahwash, MD
Associate Professor in Internal Medicine
Division of Cardiovascular Medicine Section of Heart Failure/
    Transplant
Director of the Heart and Vascular Research Organization
The Ohio State University Wexner Medical Center
Davis Heart and Lung Research Institute
Columbus, Ohio

Ankur Kalra, MD
Cardiovascular Surgery
Houston Methodist DeBakey Heart & Vascular Center
Houston, Texas

Norihiko Kamioka, MD
Cardiology Research Fellow
Structural Heart and Valve Center
Emory University
Atlanta, Georgia

Samir R. Kapadia, MD
Professor of Medicine
Director, Catheterization Laboratory
Cleveland Clinic
Cleveland, Ohio

Ryan K. Kaple, MD
Interventional Cardiologist
Assistant Professor of Medicine
Yale–New Haven Hospital
Yale School of Medicine
New Haven, Connecticut

Judit Karacsonyi, MD
VA North Texas Healthcare System
University of Texas Southwestern Medical Center
Dallas, Texas;
Division of Invasive Cardiology
Second Department of Internal Medicine and Cardiology Center
University of Szeged
Szeged, Hungary

Marc R. Katz, MD
Professor of Surgery
Medical University of South Carolina
Charleston, South Carolina

John J. Kelly, BA
Structural Heart and Valve Center
Emory University School of Medicine
Atlanta, Georgia

Samuel Kessel, BSBME
School of Medicine
University of Virginia
Charlottesville, Virginia

Ung Kim, MD, PhD
Division of Cardiology
Yeungnam University Medical Center
Daegu, Republic of Korea

Neal S. Kleiman, MD
Loretta and Carl Davis Professor of Cardiology
Director, Cardiac Catheterization Laboratories
Houston Methodist Hospital
Houston, Texas;
Professor of Medicine
Weill Cornell Medical College
New York, New York

Thomas Knickelbine, MD
Division of Cardiovascular Surgery
Minneapolis Heart Institute
Minneapolis, Minnesota

Amar Krishnaswamy, MD
Department of Cardiovascular Medicine
The Cleveland Clinic Foundation
Cleveland, Ohio

Vibhu Kshettry, MD
Section of Cardiac Surgery
Minneapolis Heart Institute
Abbott Northwestern Hospital
Minneapolis, Minnesota

Shaw-Hua Kueh, MD
Department of Radiology
University of British Columbia
Vancouver, British Columbia, Canada

Ivandito Kuntijoro, MD
Consultant
Department of Cardiology
National University Heart Center
Singapore

Shingo Kuwata, MD
Universitäts Spital Zürich
Zürich, Switzerland

Jonathon Leipsic, MD, PhD
Department of Medical Imaging and Division of Cardiology
University of British Columbia
Vancouver, British Columbia, Canada

Stamatios Lerakis, MD
Division of Cardiology
Emory University School of Medicine
Atlanta, Georgia

John R. Lesser, MD
Director of Cardiovascular CT and MRI
Minneapolis Heart Institute
Minneapolis, Minnesota

Scott M. Lilly, MD PhD
Assistant Professor, Interventional Cardiology
Medical (Interventional) Director, Structural Heart Program
Division of Cardiovascular Medicine, Interventional Section
The Ohio State University Wexner Medical Center
Heart and Vascular Center
Columbus Ohio

D. Scott Lim, MD
Director–Advanced Cardiac Valve Center
Professor of Medicine & Pediatrics
University of Virginia
Charlottesville, Virginia

David Lin, MD
Minneapolis Heart Institute at Abbott Northwestern Hospital
Minneapolis, Minnesota

Francesco Maisano, MD
Universitäts Spital Zürich
Zürich, Switzerland

Gurdeep Mann, MD
Sidra Medical and Research Center
Doha, Qatar

Christopher Meduri, MD
Co-Medical Director
Marcus Heart Valve Center
Piedmont Heart Institute
Atlanta, Georgia

Stephanie Mick, MD
Interventional Cardiology
Cardiovascular Medicine
Cleveland Clinic
Cleveland, Ohio

Michael Mooney, MD
Senior Consulting Cardiologist
Minneapolis Heart Institute at Abbott Northwestern Hospital
Minneapolis, Minnesota

Aung Myat, MD, BSc(Hons)
Sussex Cardiac Centre
Brighton and Sussex University Hospitals
Brighton, United Kingdom

Srihari S. Naidu, MD
Director, Cardiac Catheterization Labs
Director, Hypertrophic Cardiomyopathy
Westchester Medical Center
Associate Professor of Medicine
New York Medical College
Valhalla, New York

Michael Neuss, MD
Heart Center Brandenburg in Bernau/Berlin
Medical School Brandenburg
Department of Cardiology
Bernau/Berlin, Germany

Fabian Nietlispach, MD
Universitäts Spital Zürich
Zürich, Switzerland

Mickaël Ohana, MD, PhD
Radiology Department
Nouvel Hôpital Civil
Strasbourg University Hospital
Illkirch, France

Ioannis Parastatidis, MD
Division of Cardiology
Emory University School of Medicine
Atlanta, Georgia

Tilak K.R. Pasala, MD
Division of Cardiology
North Shore Health System
Lenox Hill Heart and Vascular Institute of New York
New York, New York

Ateet Patel, MD
Division of Cardiology
Emory University School of Medicine
Atlanta, Georgia

Paul Pearson, MD, PhD
Professor of Surgery
Chief, Division of Cardiothoracic Surgery
Medical College of Wisconsin
Milwaukee, Wisconsin

Wesley R. Pedersen, MD
Senior Consulting Cardiologist
Minneapolis Heart Institute at Abbott Northwestern Hospital
Minneapolis, Minnesota

François Philippon, MD
Quebec Heart and Lung Institute
Laval University
Quebec City, Quebec, Canada

Augusto Pichard, MD
Senior Consultant Innovation and Structural Heart Disease
MedStar Washington Hospital Center
Professor of Medicine (Cardiology)
Georgetown University Medical School
Washington, District of Columbia

Anil Poulose, MD
Senior Consulting Cardiologist
Minneapolis Heart Institute
Abbott Northwestern Hospital
Minneapolis, Minnesota

Alberto Pozzoli, MD
Universitäts Spital Zürich
Zürich, Switzerland

Matthew J. Price, MD
Director, Cardiac Catheterization Laboratory
Division of Cardiovascular Diseases
Scripps Clinic
La Jolla, California

Vivek Rajagopal, MD
Co-Medical Director
Marcus Heart Valve Center
Piedmont Heart Institute
Atlanta, Georgia

Claire Raphael, MBBS, PhD
Advanced Interventional Fellow
Department of Cardiovascular Medicine
Mayo Clinic
Rochester, Minnesota

Michael J. Reardon, MD
Professor of Cardiothoracic Surgery
Allison Family Distinguished Chair of Cardiovascular Research
Houston Methodist Hospital
Department of Cardiovascular Surgery
Houston, Texas

Evelyn Regar, MD
Universitäts Spital Zürich
Zürich, Switzerland

Josep Rodés-Cabau, MD
Cardiology
Quebec Heart and Lung Institute
Quebec, Canada

Jason H. Rogers, MD
Professor, Cardiovascular Medicine
Director, Interventional Cardiology
University of California, Davis Medical Center
Sacramento, California

Carlos E. Ruiz, MD, PhD
Director, Structural and Congenital Heart Center
Hackensack University Medical Center
Professor of Cardiology in Pediatrics and Medicine
The Joseph M. Sanzari Children's Hospital
Hackensack University–School of Medicine
Hackensack, New Jersey

Michael Salinger, MD
Director, Cardiac Structural Interventions
Froedtert Memorial Lutheran Hospital
Professor of Medicine and Surgery
Medical College of Wisconsin
Milwaukee, Wisconsin

Muhamed Saric, MD, PhD
Associate Professor, Department of Medicine
Clinical Director, Non-Invasive Cardiology
New York University Langone Medical Center
New York, New York

Lowell Satler, MD
Medical Director
Cardiovascular Training and Educational Center
Director of Coronary Interventions
MedStar Washington Hospital Center
Washington, District of Columbia

Jacqueline Saw, MD, FRCPC
Clinical Professor
Vancouver General Hospital
University of British Columbia
Vancouver, British Columbia, Canada

Lynelle Schneider, PA-C
The Minneapolis Heart Institute
Abbott Northwestern Hospital
Minneapolis, Minnesota

Atman P. Shah, MD
Section of Cardiology
Department of Medicine
The University of Chicago
Chicago, Illinois

Rahul Sharma, MD
Swedish Heart and Vascular
Seattle, Washington

Mark Victor Sherrid, MD
Director, Hypertrophic Cardiomyopathy Program
Professor of Medicine
Department of Medicine
New York University Langone Medical Center
New York, New York

Joy S. Shome, MBBS, MRCP
Division of Imaging Sciences and Biomedical Engineering
King's College London, Guy's and St. Thomas' Hospitals
London, United Kingdom

Horst Sievert, MD, PhD
Cardiovascular Center Frankfurt
Frankfurt, Germany

Gagan D. Singh, MD
Assistant Professor
Cardiovascular Medicine
University of California, Davis Medical Center
Sacramento, California

Thomas W. Smith, MD
Associate Clinical Professor
Division of Cardiovascular Medicine
University of California, Davis
Sacramento, California

Benjamin Sun, MD
Section of Cardiac Surgery
Minneapolis Heart Institute
Abbott Northwestern Hospital
Minneapolis, Minnesota

Hussam Suradi, MD
Director, Structural Heart & Valve Center
Interventional Cardiology
Community Hospital
Munster, Indiana;
Assistant Professor of Internal Medicine & Pediatrics
Rush University Medical Center
Chicago, Illinois

Gilbert H. L. Tang, MD, MSc, MBA
Associate Professor
Cardiovascular Surgery
Mount Sinai Medical Center
New York, New York

Maurizio Taramasso, MD
Universitäts Spital Zürich
Zürich, Switzerland

Jay Thakkar, MD
Vancouver General Hospital
Vancouver, British Columbia, Canada

Vinod H. Thourani, MD
Professor of Surgery
Cardiac Surgery
MedStar Heart and Vascular Institute/Georgetown University
Washington, District of Columbia

Stacey Tonne, BS, CVT
Minneapolis Heart Institute at Abbott Northwestern Hospital
Minneapolis, Minnesota

Imre Ungi, MD, PhD
Division of Invasive Cardiology
Second Department of Internal Medicine and Cardiology Center
University of Szeged
Szeged, Hungary

Laura Vaskelyte, MD
Cardiovascular Center Frankfurt
Frankfurt, Germany

Joseph M. Venturini, MD
Section of Cardiology
Department of Medicine
The University of Chicago
Chicago, Illinois

Marko Vezmar, MD
Pediatric Cardiologist
The Children's Heart Clinic
Minneapolis, Minnesota

Ron Waksman, MD
Director
MedStar Cardiovascular Research Network
MedStar Washington Hospital Center
Washington, District of Columbia

Zuyue Wang, MD
MedStar Cardiovascular Research Network
MedStar Washington Hospital Center
Washington, District of Columbia

John Graydon Webb, MD
Director, Interventional Cardiology
St. Paul's Hospital
McLeod Professor of Heart Valve Innovation
University of British Columbia
Medical Director, Transcatheter Valve Program
Province of British Columbia
Vancouver, British Columbia, Canada

Dominik M. Wiktor, MD
Assistant Professor of Medicine
Structural and Congenital Cardiac Interventions
University of Colorado School of Medicine
Aurora, Colorado

Mathew R. Williams, MD
Assistant Professor
Department of Surgery and Medicine
Columbia Medical Center
New York, New York

Preface

The evolution of transcatheter therapy for patients with structural heart disease has been nothing short of extraordinary. Therapies that previously required open surgery now can be done with minimally-invasive approaches that significantly improve the morbidity and longevity of many patients' lives. Nonetheless, these techniques can be complex, difficult to describe, and challenging to apply. These issues are especially germane as formal training programs in structural heart interventions are relatively few and, even if undertaken, can be limited in scope.

In this atlas, we describe essential and innovative transcatheter techniques for treating these patients with a case-based, pithy format, which emphasizes key learnings. Some techniques are unique. Others, such as the creation of exteriorized rails and advanced imaging, share common features and can serve as the foundation for many transcatheter approaches. Potential hazards and learnings for their future avoidance are essential for all practitioners and also are an important focus of this atlas. The descriptions and illustrations of these clinical pearls and pitfalls serve to enhance the expertise for all persons who evaluate and treat patients with structural heart disease.

Undoubtedly, transcatheter therapy for patients with structural heart disease will continue to evolve rapidly. Our field was founded on the creativity and courage of many pioneers, their staff, and their patients. The evolution of the field requires that we continue to explore and test the boundaries for what is possible. The essential goals of our profession, which are represented in this atlas, are to address unmet clinical needs, improve the health of our patients, and educate others so that many more lives will benefit.

Acknowledgements

This book was made possible only with the wonderful contributions of all of the authors and the work of their medical teams, and the privileges given to us all by the patients who entrust us with their lives. I am indebted to many teachers who have inspired a love of science and medicine and a passion for education. Professional success is rare without mentorship, and I am particularly indebted to Dr. Rick A. Nishimura, who has been a special mentor to me for decades.

I also would like to especially acknowledge the support of my colleagues at the Minneapolis Heart Institute at Abbott Northwestern Hospital, Allina Health, and the Valve Science Center at the Minneapolis Heart Institute Foundation. Their support and trust in our care enabled many of the innovations described in this book, and their tireless work continues to bring state-of-the-art, exemplary care to many patients in need.

Contents

Mitral Valve Disease

Uncomplicated Transcatheter Mitral Valve Repair With MitraClip

Paul Sorajja, MD

A 91-year-old man with multiple morbidities and prohibitive surgical risk was referred for transcatheter repair with Mitra-Clip (Abbott Vascular, Santa Clara, CA).

A, On transesophageal echocardiography (TEE), there was degenerative mitral regurgitation (MR) with a small flail segment (arrowhead). B, Severe MR was present on color flow imaging (arrow). C, On the TEE bi-commissural view, the flail segment arose slightly medial (arrowhead). D, Transseptal puncture is performed at a height of 3.9 cm to the mitral coaptation point. For the classic MitraClip system, a transseptal height of ~4.0 cm was sufficient, but a height of ~4.5 cm is typically used for MitraClip NT. E, The clip delivery system (CDS) is inserted into the steerable guide catheter (SGC) and straddled. Arrowheads indicate straddle markers; arrow indicates SGC tip. F, The CDS is steered toward the mitral valve using the M knob and posterior torque of the SGC, followed by opening of the clip arms. G, TEE with 3-dimensional imaging allows the clip arms to be centered over the target of pathology; the arms are positioned perpendicular to the coaptation plane of the mitral valve. H, The CDS crosses the mitral valve, followed by closure of the arms to 120 degrees to enable cupping of the leaflets. I, Once the leaflets fall into the arms, the grippers are dropped and the arms are closed to 60 degrees. Leaflet insertion is confirmed in multiple views. J, The clip then is completely closed, followed by an assessment for MR reduction. This closure is preferably done in the bi-commissural view with simultaneous color imaging to show the location of the clip and effect on MR reduction. K, The mitral gradient is checked for possible stenosis. L, TEE imaging shows trivial residual MR after final clip deployment.

Ao, Ascending aorta; L, lateral; LA, left atrium; LV, left ventricle; M, medial; RA, right atrium; RV, right ventricle.

KEY POINTS

- In experienced centers, transcatheter mitral valve repair with MitraClip is an effective and safe procedure for the treatment of severe, symptomatic MR.

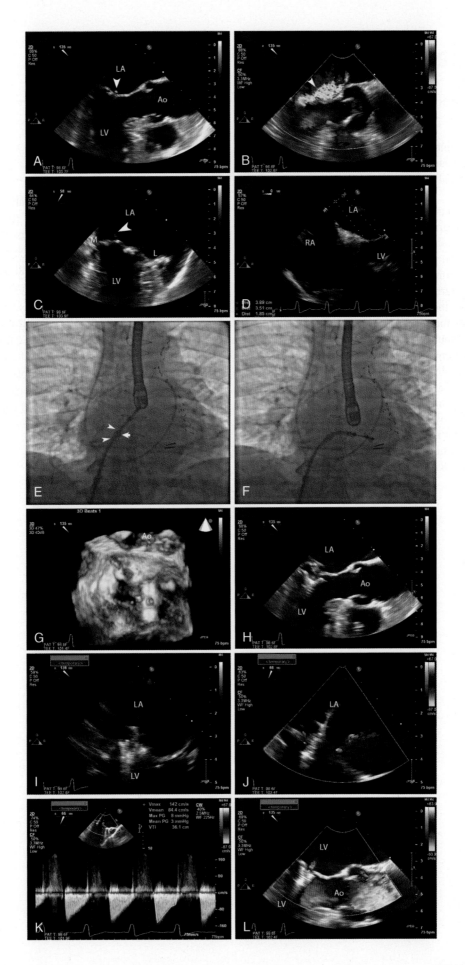

Commissural Mitral Regurgitation Therapy

Paul Sorajja, MD

An 87-year-old woman with multiple morbidities was referred for transcatheter treatment of symptomatic, severe mitral regurgitation (MR) with MitraClip (Abbott Vascular, Santa Clara, CA).

A and B, Left ventricular outflow tract view on transesophageal echocardiography (TEE) demonstrates fibroelastic deficiency of the mitral valve and severe MR (arrowheads). C and D, Commissural imaging shows a flail segment on the medial side of the mitral valve, in association with MR on color flow-imaging (arrowheads). E, For effective grasping of the mitral leaflets, the clip arms should be placed perpendicular to the coaptation plane of the valve. For medial jets, the arms therefore should be rotated counterclockwise, often ending up in the region of 11 and 5 o'clock on a clock face. F, Placement of the clip here leads to significant reduction in MR. G, TEE with 3-dimensional imaging shows a large single orifice of the mitral valve (asterisk). H, TEE with color-flow imaging shows the final result with elimination of the MR following clip release.

Ao, Ascending aorta; L, lateral; LA, left atrium; LV, left ventricle; M, medial; RA, right atrium; RV, right ventricle.

KEY POINTS

- In patients with commissural MR, the clip arms of the MitraClip device must be rotated to become perpendicular to the mitral coaptation plane for leaflet grasping. Placement of clips in the commissures will result in asymmetrical double-orifices or even a single-orifice, and such asymmetry has no clinical relevance.
- Chordal entanglement is a hazard when maneuvering the MitraClip in the commissures. This risk is minimized through careful alignment of the clip arms above the annular plane, and minimizing catheter rotation once the clip arms cross the mitral valve leaflets into the left ventricle.

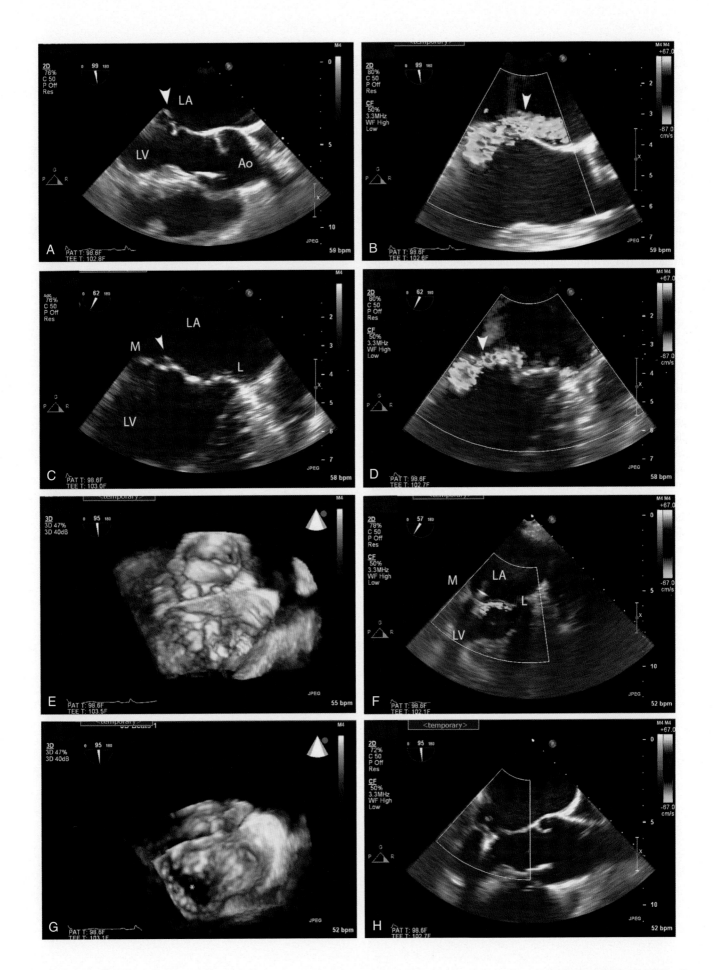

Advanced Steering in the Left Atrium for an Aortic Hugger

Mario Gössl, MD, PhD

The preferred location for the transseptal puncture in a Mitra-Clip procedure is posterior and at the level of the medial commissure of the mitral valve. Some punctures, however, may occur too anteriorly. As a result, considerable difficulty with leaflet grasping arises because the trajectory of the steerable sleeve is anterior-to-posterior (A, arrow; G, arrow), and thus not perpendicular to the mitral annular plane ("aorta hugger"). (B) Without perpendicularity, simultaneous grasping of both leaflets is challenging, particularly when there is a large gap height, markedly asymmetrical leaflet lengths, or mitral annular calcification present. When an aorta hugger occurs, inadequate grasping of the anterior leaflet can be difficult (B, arrow).

Common causes for this scenario are slippage of the transseptal needle during advancement (typically superior from the intended puncture site) or travel through a patent foramen ovale. The transseptal puncture may be repeated to gain a relatively posterior position, or the following advanced steering maneuver can be utilized: (C) Model of the mitral valve (MV) and interatrial septum (IAS) that illustrates the trajectory of the aorta hugger, which travels posterior to anterior in the apical direction. (D) To counter the effect of the aorta hugger, "+" is added to the steerable guide catheter (arrow), leading to posterior movement of the steerable sleeve (arrowheads). (E) Next, "A" is added to the sleeve leading to antero-lateral trajectory (arrowheads). (F) "M" is

then applied to center the sleeve in the middle of the MV. (H) Repeat three-dimensional echocardiography showing improvement in the trajectory following the previous maneuvers (arrowheads).

Ao, Ascending aorta; Ant, anterior; IAS, interatrial septum; LA, left atrium; LV, left ventricle; M, medial; MV, mitral valve; Post, posterior.

KEY POINTS

- Stay posterior and avoid aiming anteriorly during the transeptal puncture.
- Without perpendicularity, simultaneous grasping of both leaflets is challenging, particularly when there is a large gap height, markedly asymmetrical leaflet lengths, or mitral annular calcification present.
- When an aorta hugger is encountered, apply "+" to the steerable guiding catheter, followed by "A" and "M" on the steerable sleeve. These advanced maneuvers will stand the steerable sleeve up and allow for a more perpendicular position of the MitraClip to the mitral annular plane.

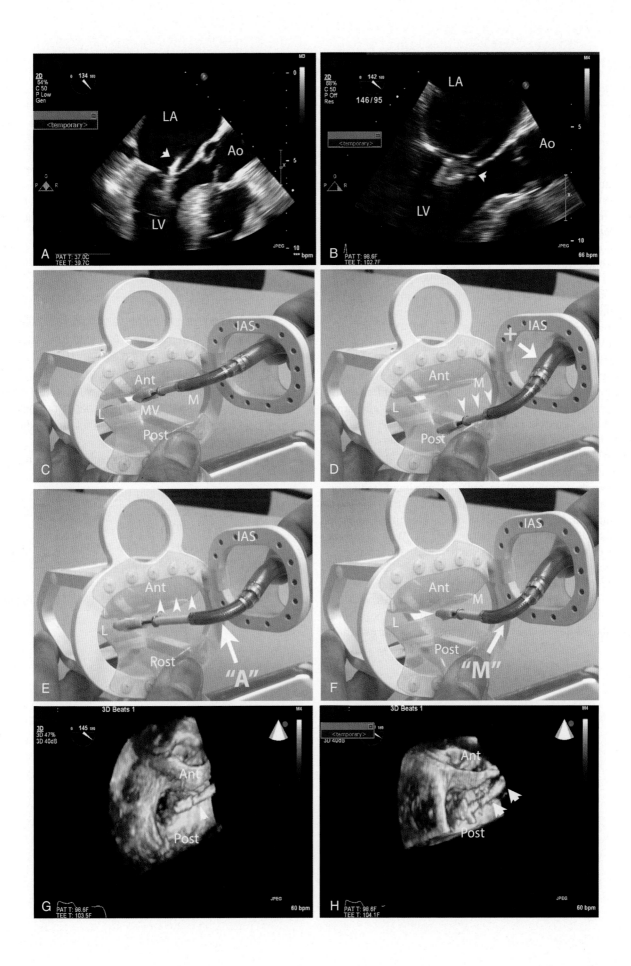

Transcatheter Repair of Ruptured Papillary Muscle

Paul Sorajja, MD, David Lin, MD, Judah Askew, MD, and Michael Mooney, MD

An 85-year-old man with severe aortic stenosis underwent transcatheter, transapical placement of a 26 mm Sapien S3 prosthesis. Following aortic valve replacement, new, severe mitral regurgitation (MR) occurred due to rupture of the anterolateral papillary muscle. Due to his prohibitive surgical risk, he underwent emergent transcatheter repair with Mitra-Clip (Abbott Vascular, Santa Clara, CA).

A, Transesophageal echocardiography (TEE) demonstrates severe MR (arrowhead). Imaging with TEE shows the ruptured papillary muscle in the left atrium in systole (B, arrow) and in the left ventricle in diastole (C, arrow). D, A relatively low mitral height (4.0 cm) was chosen for the transseptal puncture given the lateral location of the mitral pathology. E, With slight counterclockwise rotation, the clip arms are aligned perpendicular to the lateral mitral coaptation plane (arrow). F, With introduction of the clip arms into the left ventricle (arrows), movement of the papillary muscle in and out of the left atrium continues (arrowheads). G, With appropriate timing, the grippers are dropped to grasp the mitral leaflets to trap the ruptured papillary muscle in the left ventricle (arrowhead) in order to maximize reduction in MR as seen in this left ventricular outflow tract view. H, Bi-commissural imaging also shows the papillary muscle trapped in the left ventricle (arrowhead). I, With complete closure of the clip arms, the diastolic mitral gradient is prohibitively high at 19 mm Hg. J, With opening of the clip arms to 30 degrees, the mitral gradient is reduced to 7 mm Hg. K and L, Multiple views show only mild residual MR with the clip arms open at 30 degrees (arrowheads). M, Fluoroscopy shows the 30-degree final arm angle for the clip (arrowhead).

N, The final arm angle is established, followed by release of the clip (arrowhead).

Ao Ascending aorta; Av, aortic valve prosthesis; LA, left atrium; LV, left ventricle; RA, right atrium; RV, right ventricle; SGC, steerable guide catheter.

KEY POINTS

- Entanglement of the mitral valve apparatus during transcatheter aortic therapy can lead to disruption of the papillary muscles and severe MR.
- A ruptured papillary muscle can be effectively treated with transcatheter mitral valve repair with MitraClip. Ideally the ruptured papillary muscle should be trapped in the left ventricle to maximize reduction of MR.
- Due to the acute nature of the pathology, the mitral annulus may be relatively small and lead to high mitral gradients with clip deployment. These gradients can be minimized with slight opening of the clip arms (up to 30 degrees).
- When leaving the clip arms slightly open during deployment, the final arm angle should be well visualized on fluoroscopy and established with routine measures before final release of the gripper line.

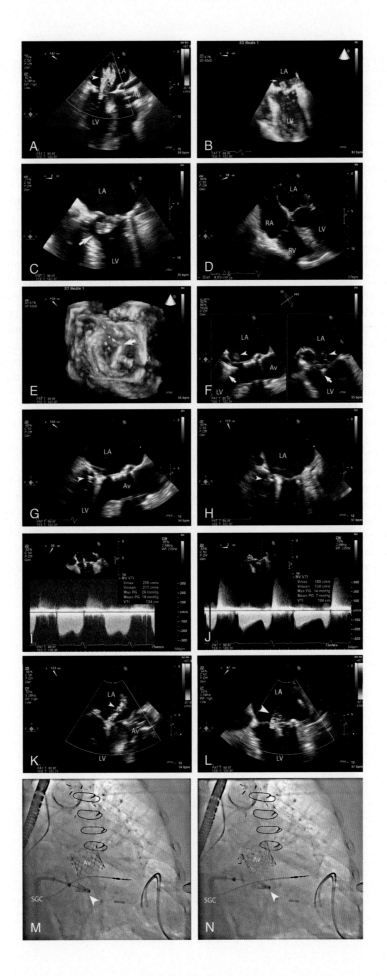

Optimal Intraprocedural Guidance for Mitral Therapy

Richard Bae, MD, and Paul Sorajja, MD

Transesophageal echocardiography (TEE) is essential for guiding transcatheter mitral valve (MV) therapy, such as MitraClip (Abbott Vascular, Santa Clara, CA). A–F, Imaging guidance for the transseptal puncture (arrowheads). A, Bicaval view showing superior and inferior trajectory of the puncture. B, Short-axis view of the aortic valve and atrial septum, showing anterior-posterior trajectory. The puncture site is posteriorly located. C, Four-chamber view for measurement of distance or height of the puncture to the mitral annular plane. D, Reverse four-chamber view for confirmatory check of the puncture height. E and F, Using TEE, 3-dimensional views of the fossa (F) and mitral annular plane confirm the trajectory and puncture location relative to the medial commissure. G–I, The clip arms must be oriented perpendicular to the mitral coaptation plane. G, 3-D view showing orientation of the clip arms (arrowhead) to be perpendicular relative to the mitral coaptation plane when positioned in the left atrium above the MV. H, Following advancement of the clip into the left ventricle, 3-D viewing with a decrease in the gain allows imaging of the clip arms, and indicates their orientation (arrowhead) without the need for transgastric viewing. On this image, the clip arms (arrowhead) are incorrectly rotated. I, With clockwise rotation, the clip arms (arrowhead) are correctly rotated to be perpendicular to the mitral coaptation plane. J, X-plane imaging confirms the clips are equally viewed in the left ventricular outflow tract view (right panel) and appropriately not visible on the orthogonal, commissural view (left panel).

K–N, "Aortic hugger" imaging. K, In situations where the transseptal puncture is too low or too anterior, the trajectory of the clip delivery system (arrowhead) will pose challenges for grasping the anterior and posterior leaflets together or equally. L, This unfavorable trajectory can be seen easily with 3-D, side-imaging of the clip delivery system relative to the MV plane (arrow). M, Following addition of "plus" on the guide and "A" on the steerable sleeve, the aortic hugger is corrected and the imaging confirms a more appropriate trajectory (arrow). N, This correction and the more favorable trajectory is also seen on 2-dimensional imaging (arrow).

Ao, Ascending aorta; IAS, interatrial septum; LA, left atrium; LV, left ventricle; MV mitral valve; RA, right atrium; RV, right ventricle; SVC, superior vena cava.

KEY POINTS

- Tranesophageal imaging is essential for guidance transcatheter MV repair. Goals of the imaging include indicating the appropriate transseptal puncture location (posterior with adequate height to the MV), orientation of the clip arms relative to the mitral coaptation plane, and assisting with trajectory of the steerable sleeve.

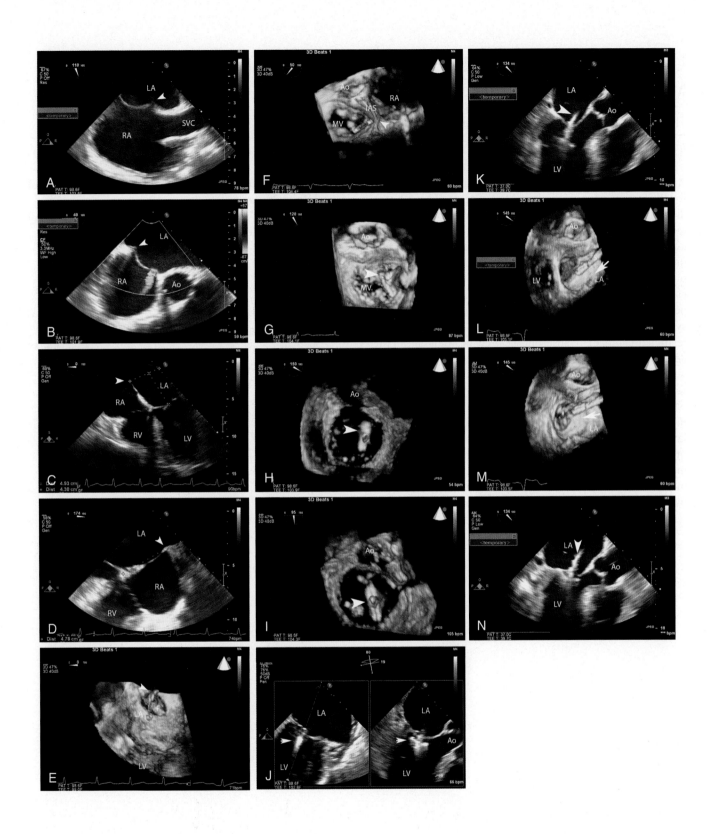

Challenges of Transcatheter Therapy for Functional Mitral Regurgitation

Thomas W. Smith, MD, Gagan Singh, MD, and Jason H. Rogers, MD

A 78-year-old man with progressive dyspnea was referred for evaluation of mitral valve (MV) disease. The echocardiogram demonstrated a dilated left ventricle with severely reduced systolic function and severe functional mitral regurgitation (MR). MR remained severe despite maximal medical therapy. After evaluation by a cardiothoracic surgeon and a multidisciplinary heart team, he was considered to be a poor candidate for surgical MV intervention, and was referred for percutaneous transcatheter valve repair with the MitraClip system (Abbott Vascular, Santa Clara, CA). A and B (arrow, restricted chordae), Transesophageal echocardiogram (TEE) demonstrated restricted anterior and posterior mitral leaflets with severe central regurgitation. C, An initial grasp was performed on the medial aspect of the severe jet (medial A2:P2) with modest MR reduction. D, A second clip was then placed in the central portion of the jet, with distortion of the more lateral orifice zone of coaptation and significant worsening of the MR laterally. E, The central clip was released and moved laterally to the lateral edge of A2:P2, resulting in a more favorable coaptation zone with significant reduction in overall MR. The patient was discharged, and did well with a reduction in MR to 1+, and a mean diastolic MV gradient of 5 mm Hg at 30-day follow-up.

Ao, Ascending aorta; LA, left atrium; Lat, lateral; LV, left ventricle; Med, medial.

KEY POINTS

- In functional mitral regurgitation with restricted leaflets, each MitraClip placement may alter the adjacent coaptation zone and affect severity of regurgitation.
- Careful TEE assessment following each MitraClip grasp is essential to evaluate for unexpected valve conformation changes.
- Consider a triple orifice MV repair (one MitraClip medial and one lateral), if there is inadequate reduction in MR with a central grasp.

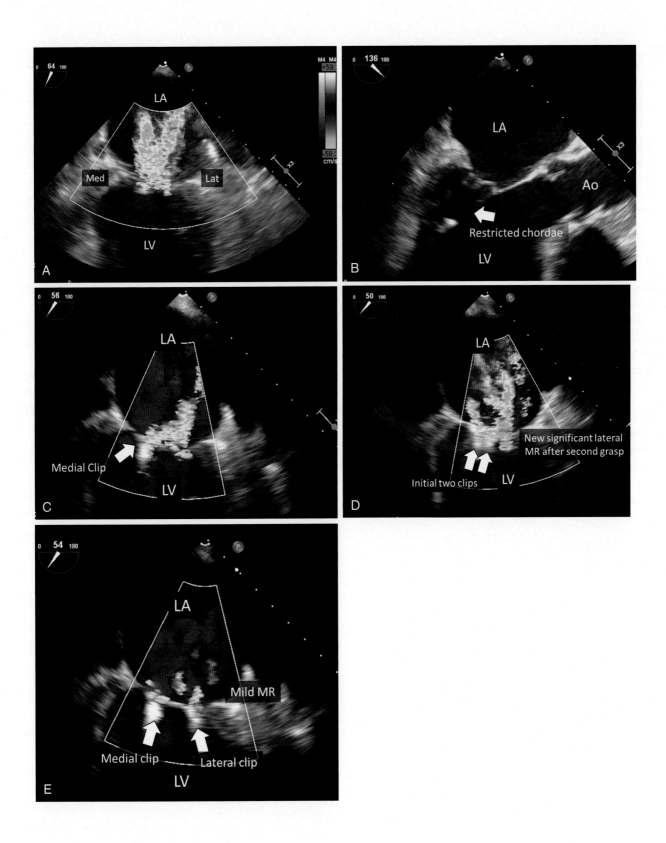

The Zip-and-Clip Technique in Transcatheter Mitral Valve Repair

Paul Sorajja, MD

A 90-year-old woman with severe symptomatic mitral regurgitation (MR) and prohibitive surgical risk was referred for transcatheter mitral valve repair with MitraClip (Abbott Vascular, Santa Clara, CA). A, On transesophageal echocardiography (TEE), there was a large flail gap (arrow) due to multiple ruptured chords. B, Severe MR in association with this flail segment was present (arrowhead). C, The predominant jet of MR was lateral on TEE imaging with a bi-commissural view. Multiple attempts at grasping the lateral segments were unsuccessful. D, A grasp medial to the target location was then performed (arrow). This placement did not alter the degree of MR (arrowhead). E, However, the medial grasp brought the lateral segments (arrowhead) closer together (i.e., "bunching" or "zipping"), thereby reducing the gap height and enabling additional clipping to be performed. F, Residual MR with third clip in place is trivial on imaging with bi-commissural views. G, TEE with 3-dimensional imaging showing the tissue bridge created from placement of three clips. H, Final echocardiographic result with color compare imaging shows trivial residual MR.

Ao, Ascending aorta; L, lateral; LA, left atrium; LV, left ventricle.

KEY POINTS

- The "zip-and-clip" maneuver is a technique to address large gap heights for patients undergoing transcatheter mitral valve repair with MitraClip.
- In this technique, the initial clip placed may or may not affect MR, and the operator needs to be confident that the placement of the initial clip reduces the gap height for additional clipping.
- "Zipping" is preferably performed by starting in the commissures and working toward the central, chord-free zone of the mitral valve.
- As for all patients undergoing multiple clipping, adequate room must be made available for all of the clips without concern for causing significant mitral stenosis.

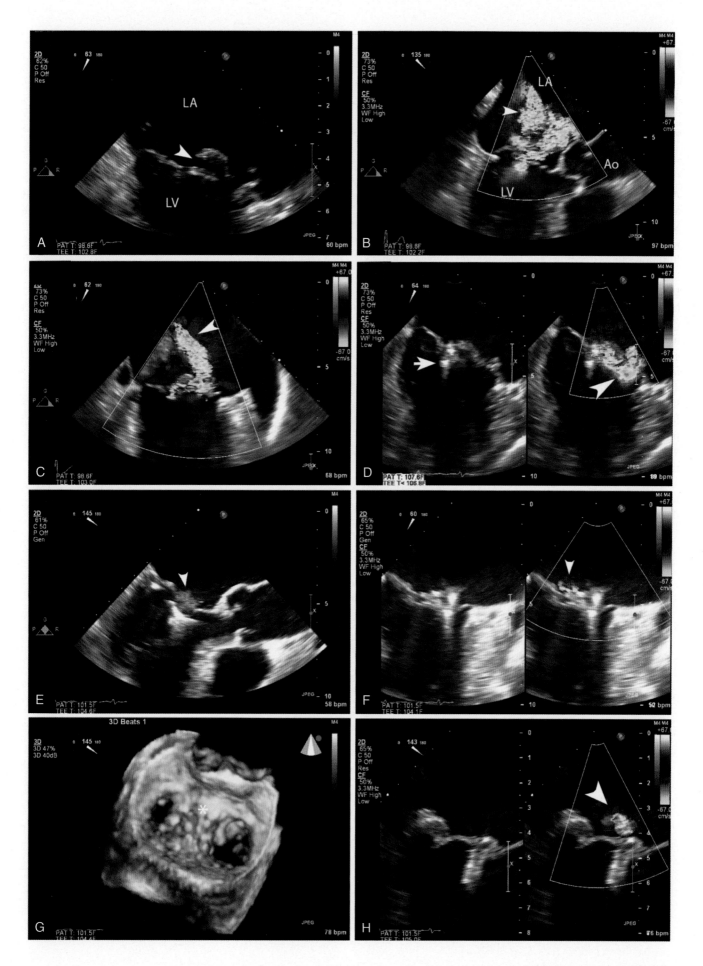

Mitral Annular Calcification and Transcatheter Mitral Valve Repair

Paul Sorajja, MD

A 90-year-old woman was referred for treatment of symptomatic mitral regurgitation (MR) with MitraClip (Abbott Vascular, Santa Clara, CA). Her medical history was significant for chronic renal insufficiency (estimated glomerular filtration rate, 32 cc/min) and long-standing hypertension.

A, Transesophageal echocardiography (TEE) demonstrated a torn chord involving the posterior mitral leaflet (arrow), with significant posterior mitral annular calcification (MAC, arrowhead). B, The MAC, which is present along much of the posterior annulus, is visible on 3-dimensional echocardiography in a surgeon's view (arrowheads). The mean mitral gradient was only 1 mm Hg (not shown). C, To maximize the ability to maneuver the steerable sleeve of the clip delivery system around the MAC, the most posterior location possible is chosen for the transseptal puncture. This posterior location is best seen on short-axis view of the aortic valve with TEE (arrowhead). The height of the puncture to the mitral valve was 4.7 cm (not shown). D, The steerable sleeve is positioned considerably posterior (arrowhead) to the aorta, and the clip arm is able to be placed between the MAC and the posterior mitral leaflet. E, Following clip deployment, the flail segment is treated and the residual MR is mild. F, TEE with 3-dimensional imaging showing the tissue bridge created with clip deployment (arrow).

Ao, Ascending aorta; LA, left atrium; LV, left ventricle; RA, right atrium.

KEY POINTS

- For patients with mitral annular calcification, transcatheter repair of MR can be performed with MitraClip. The mitral valve area should be suitable to accommodate clip placement without significant stenosis.
- A markedly posterior transseptal puncture facilitates maneuvering of the steerable sleeve of the MitraClip around MAC for treatment of MR.

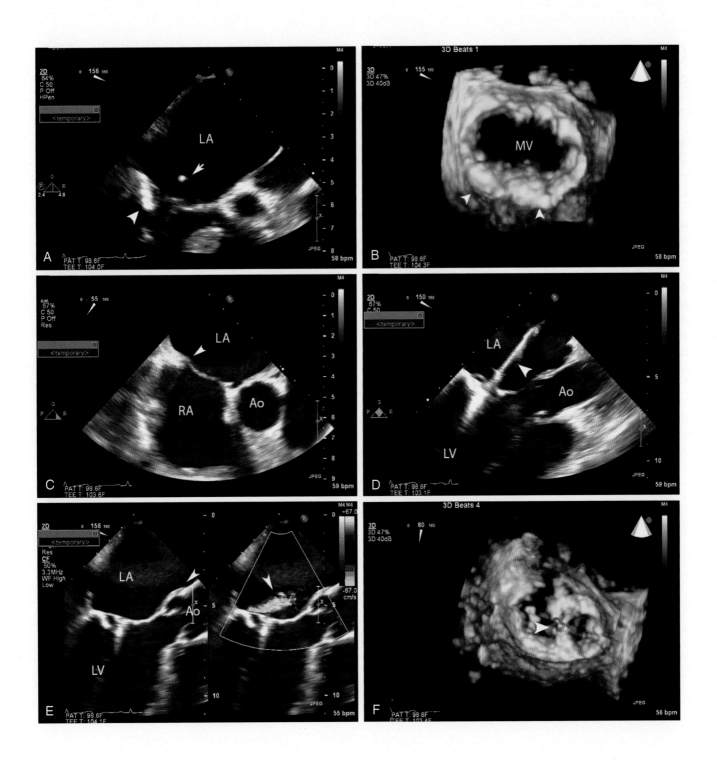

Optimization of Multiple Clip Placement

Paul Sorajja, MD

An 83-year-old man with severe degenerative mitral regurgitation (MR) and multiple morbidities is referred for transcatheter repair with MitraClip (Abbott Vascular, Santa Clara, CA).

A, Baseline transesophageal echocardiogram showing severe MR on color-flow imaging (arrowhead). B, A clip is placed at the site of the MR with proper leaflet insertion. C, Following initial placement (arrow), there continues to be significant MR with regurgitation occurring on both sides of the clip. D, The clip is moved medially (arrowhead), leaving adequate room for a second clip in the A2-P2 segments of the mitral valve (MV) to treat the residual regurgitation. E, A second clip is placed (arrow) lateral to the first one (arrowhead). F, Mild residual MR is present following placement of two clips.

Ao, Ascending aorta; L, lateral; LA, left atrium; LV, left ventricle; M, medial.

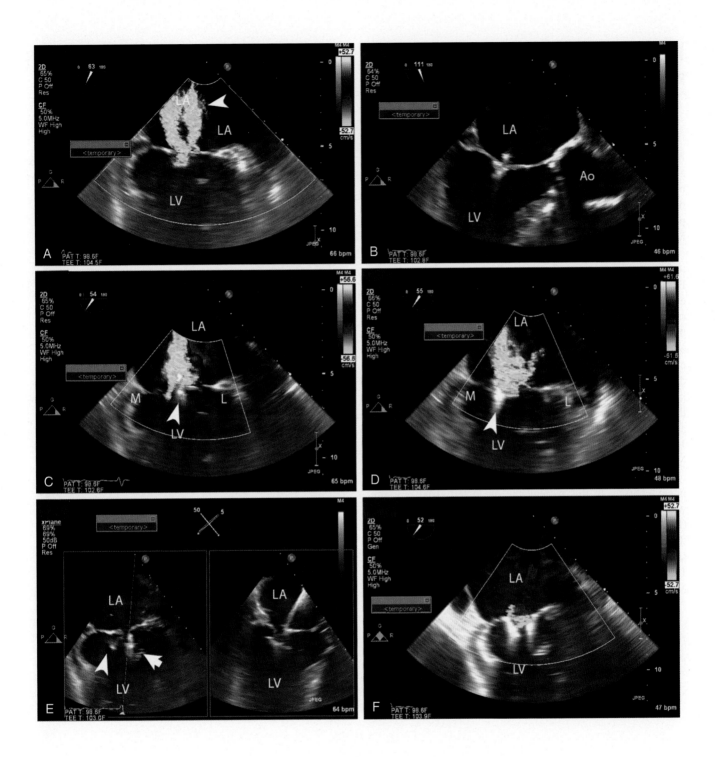

Importance of Hemodynamics for Assessing Residual Regurgitation

Paul Sorajja, MD

An 84-year-old man was referred for treatment of symptomatic, severe mitral regurgitation (MR), in the setting of multiple, high-risk morbidities (for example, prior stroke, chronic renal failure, and frailty). His MR was primarily due to a flail posterior leaflet, and he underwent transcatheter repair with MitraClip (Abbott Vascular, Santa Clara, CA).

A, Transesophageal echocardiogram showing a flail posterior mitral leaflet involving the P2 segment (arrowhead). B, The flail segment is also easily visible on 3-dimensional echocardiography of mitral valve (MV) in a surgeon's view (arrowhead). C, A single clip (arrowhead) is placed to target the flail portion, leading to apposition of the A2-P2 segments of the MV. D, Residual MR is present after placement of clip despite treatment of the flail segment. On some echocardiography views, the residual MR appears to be more than mild (arrowhead). E and F, Prior to placing a second clip, the left atrial pressures are examined. In our practice, the left atrial pressure is examined at a systolic blood pressure of 150 mm Hg to gain insight into the dynamic nature of the MR and volume overload prior to MitraClip therapy. This hemodyanamic study frequently requires administration of phenylephrine. In this patient, the mean left atrial pressure was 38 mm Hg at a systolic blood pressure of 147 mm Hg (E). Following placement of the clip, re-examination of the hemodynamics shows that the mean left atrial pressure is now only 13 mm Hg at a systolic blood pressure of 152 mm Hg (F). This finding demonstrates that the residual MR is not associated with significant left atrial hypertension at rest or during dynamic maneuvers. A second clip therefore was not placed, and the patient did well with no symptoms in follow-up.

Ao, Ascending aorta; LA, left atrium; LV, left ventricle.

KEY POINTS

- MR and its effects on left atrial hypertension are highly dynamic.
- Examining left atrial pressure at rest and under provocation (that is, hypertension) provides incremental utility, in addition to comprehensive echocardiography, for determining the clinical importance of residual MR with MitraClip therapy.
- Measurement of left atrial pressure with provocation should be assessed before and after clip placement to help determine effectiveness of the procedure.
- Inadequate reduction in left atrial pressure may occur with incomplete treatment of MR, iatrogenic mitral stenosis, excessive fluid administration during the procedure (for example, anesthetic administration or turning up the drips for clip detachment), or significant diastolic dysfunction.

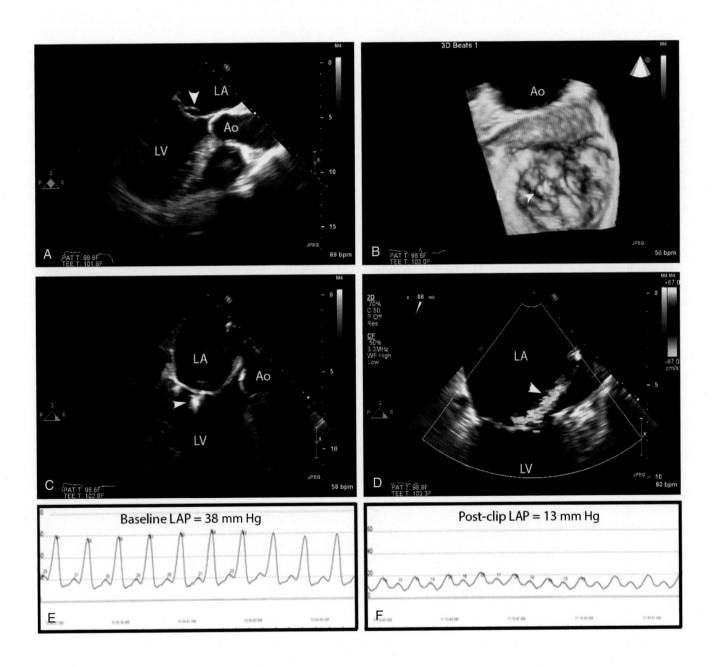

Use of Low-Profile Catheter for Continuous Left Atrial Pressure Monitoring During Transcatheter Mitral Valve Repair

Claire E. Raphael, MD, and Mackram F. Eleid, MD

An 88-year-old woman with severe mitral regurgitation (MR) was hospitalized with pulmonary edema. She had a history of coronary artery disease, acute on chronic renal failure, atrial fibrillation, and morbid obesity. Surgical mitral valve (MV) repair was not possible due to prohibitive risk. Transesophageal echocardiography (TEE) revealed severe, eccentric MR secondary to a flail P2 posterior leaflet (C). Transcatheter MV repair with MitraClip (Abbott Vascular, Santa Clara, CA) was performed under general anesthesia with TEE guidance. Transseptal puncture was performed in a superior-posterior position. A 4F multipurpose catheter was inserted in the right superior pulmonary vein for continuous pressure monitoring. A, The 24-Fr MitraClip steerable guide catheter was placed in the left atrium (LA). B, MitraClips were positioned under TEE guidance. D, The first clip was placed laterally, and resulted in improvement in MR, and a reduction of the LA v-wave from 50 mm Hg to 35 mm Hg;

however, a medial jet of MR remained, consistent with the persistent elevation in the v-wave. E, A second clip was placed medially, and further reduction of the LA v-wave to 18 mm Hg occurred. The residual MR was only mild.

KEY POINTS

- A 4F multipurpose catheter can be safely positioned in the pulmonary vein and does not interfere with MitraClip insertion.
- Continuous LA pressure monitoring during MitraClip therapy gives complementary information to the TEE, and helps to guide intraprocedural decision making.

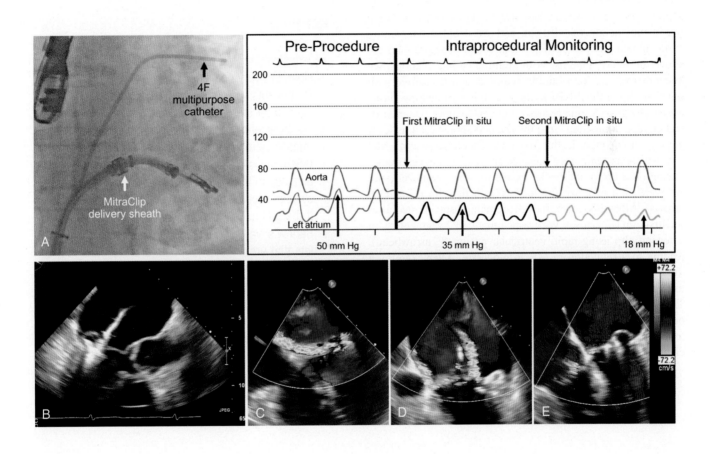

Barlow's Valve Therapy

Christopher Meduri, MD, and Vivek Rajagopal, MD

A 67-year-old man with severe symptoms from mitral regurgitation (MR) secondary to Barlow's disease was evaluated. On transesophageal echocardiography, there was a flail leaflet (A, arrowhead) with severe MR (B, arrows). Because of impaired mobility due to Parkinson's disease, our heart team deemed him to be extreme surgical risk, and we elected to proceed with transcatheter mitral valve (MV) repair using the MitraClip system (Abbott Vascular, Santa Clara, CA). There was a flail height of ~1.0 cm, and we decided on gaining extra "height" by performing a transseptal puncture ~4.5 cm above the mitral annulus. With multiple flailing scallops, we knew that three clips would be required, and we started with our first clip at the A1-P1 scallops as this area had the shortest flail height. Despite numerous grasp attempts, the anterior leaflet kept "knuckling" into the grippers, preventing us from getting an adequate leaflet insertion. Therefore, we inserted a transvenous temporary pacemaker. With rapid ventricular pacing (180 bpm), the leaflet excursion was minimized, and we were able to grasp the leaflets with the clip (C and D, arrows). After this grasp, the MR remained severe medial to the first clip (E, arrow). We grasped the A2-P2 segments with a second clip using rapid ventricular pacing (F, arrowhead), leading to a reduction in MR to moderate. After examining the MV gradient (2 mm Hg), we then implanted a third clip to treat the prolapse of the A3-P3 segments (G, arrowheads). The MR was reduced to mild, and the final MV gradient was only 3 mm Hg (H, arrowhead). The patient's cardiac symptoms were significantly improved (New York Heart Association class I), although the patient remains limited by his Parkinson's disease. At one year of follow-up, all the clips remain on the leaflets with a residual MR of ≤ 2+.

A, Anterior; L, lateral; LA, left atrium; LV, left ventricle; LVOT, left ventricular outflow tract; M, medial; P, posterior; TPM, temporary pacemaker; SGC, steerable guide catheter.

KEY POINTS

- Transcatheter MV repair of Barlow's disease is feasible, but very challenging, and should be reserved for patients who are considered extreme risk candidates for surgical repair.
- Transcatheter mitral repair of Barlow's disease often requires multiple clips.
- When choosing the transseptal puncture height, the distance to the top of the mitral leaflets during their systolic excursion should be considered, especially if the gap height is significant.
- Barlow's valves have billowing, protuberant leaflets that are difficult to grasp, and rapid ventricular pacing should be considered to facilitate grasping. This redundancy can pose challenges for examination of leaflet insertion into the clip arms, which must be carefully done to minimize risk of single leaflet device attachment.

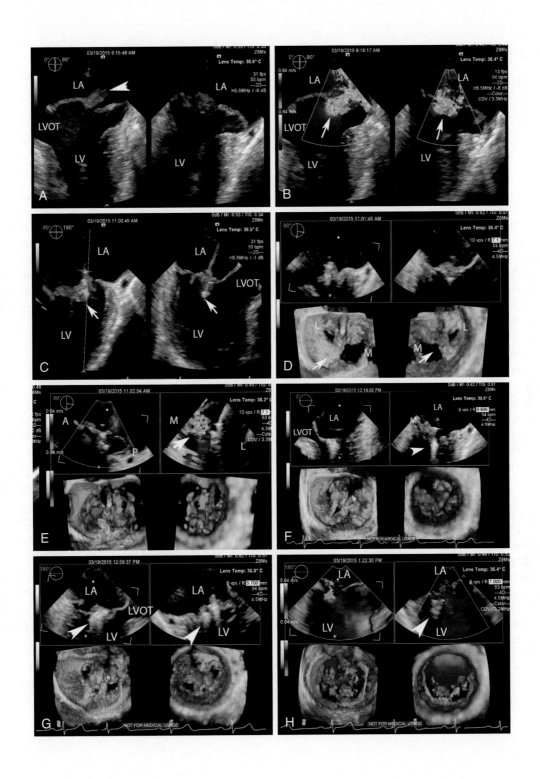

Acute Left Ventricular Dysfunction and Recovery After Transcatheter Mitral Repair

Ryan K. Kaple, MD, and Gilbert H. L. Tang, MD, MSc, MBA

A 79-year-old woman with a past medical history of dementia, frailty, low body mass index (20.6 kg/m^2), thrombocytopenia, and atrial fibrillation, presented with cardiogenic shock. She was intubated for acute hypoxic respiratory failure, initiated on inotropic support, and an intra-aortic balloon pump (IABP) was placed for hemodynamic support. Transesophageal echocardiogram (TEE) demonstrated severe mitral regurgitation (MR) due to a wide flail segment of the P2 scallop (A–C). The left ventricular ejection fraction (LVEF) was preserved at 65%, and there was moderate right ventricular dysfunction. Left heart catheterization demonstrated mild nonobstructive coronary artery disease. Right heart catheterization, performed with support from vasopressors and the IABP, showed pulmonary artery pressures of 31/19 mm Hg, pulmonary artery capillary wedge pressure of 15 mm Hg, cardiac output (CO) of 2.49 L/min, and a cardiac index of 1.61 L/min per m^2. She was deemed to be at prohibitively high risk for surgery, and thus underwent percutaneous mitral valve (MV) repair with the MitraClip system (Abbott Vascular, Santa Clara, CA). Via the traditional transseptal approach, two MitraClips were placed under TEE guidance, reducing the MR to trace-to-mild (D–F). The final mean MV gradient was 6 mm Hg. The patient was extubated immediately after the procedure. On postoperative day (POD) 1, the CO had increased to 3.6 L/min, and no inotropes were required. The IABP was subsequently removed. Four hours after IABP removal, the patient was noted to be restless and delirious, with cool extremities on exam. Transthoracic echocardiogram demonstrated an LVEF of 15% to 20%, global LV hypokinesis, moderate right ventricle (RV) dysfunction,

and mild MR. An IABP was placed and epinephrine and milrinone were initiated, with suspicion for acute afterload mismatch. The LVEF improved to 45% on POD 8, and the IABP and epinephrine were discontinued. On POD 12, the LVEF was noted to be 60%, and milrinone was discontinued. The patient was discharged to a rehabilitation center and eventually returned home. At 6-month follow-up, the echocardiogram showed an LVEF of 65%, normal RV function, and mild MR.

KEY POINTS

- High-risk surgical patients presenting with cardiogenic shock due to acute severe MR should be considered for percutaneous MV repair, either as a primary treatment or bridge to MV surgery.
- Risk factors for acute afterload mismatch following MV repair (surgical or percutaneous) or replacement include reduced LVEF and pulmonary hypertension. However, this phenomena also may occur in the absence of these risk factors.
- Acute afterload mismatch must be considered as a possible etiology for cardiogenic shock following percutaneous MV repair. Prolonged mechanical support and/or inotropes may be required to allow for recovery of ventricular function.

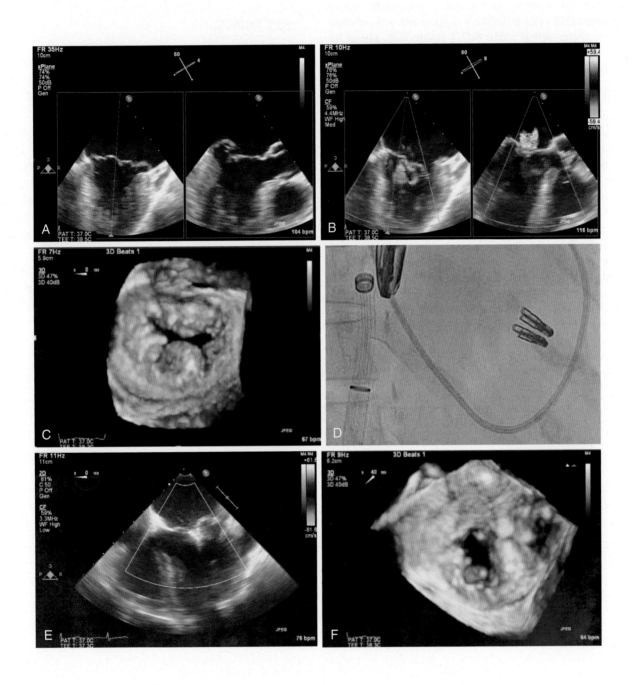

A Space Too Small for Additional Clipping

Paul Sorajja, MD

An 84-year-old woman with severe symptomatic mitral regurgitation (MR) and prohibitive surgical risk was referred for transcatheter mitral valve (MV) repair with MitraClip (Abbott Vascular, Santa Clara, CA).

A, Transesophageal echocardiography, with color-compare imaging, demonstrates severe, lateral regurgitation (arrowhead) due to primary or degenerative MR. B, 3-Dimensional (3-D) echocardiography from the left atrium (surgeon's view) shows alignment of the MitraClip along the lateral commissure of the MV (arrowhead). This position was the furthest lateral that the clip could be placed. C, Clip implantation leads to creation of a tissue bridge (arrow), with a residual lateral orifice (arrowhead). D, Significant MR through the lateral orifice (arrowhead) remains. E, An attempt to pass a second clip to the lateral orifice to treat the MR is undertaken. 3-D echocardiography shows positioning of the clip over the lateral orifice (arrow). F, The clip is advanced in a closed position and becomes caught in the mitral chords (arrow). Attempts to remove the clip with eversion, cycling of the grippers, and guide repositioning are unsuccessful. G, The second clip is then deployed in the mitral chords with persistent MR.

Ao, Ascending aorta; L, lateral; LA, left atrium; LV, left ventricle; M, medial.

KEY POINTS

- To place additional clips, there must be adequate room for passage and opening of the clip, as well as maneuvering to grasp the anterior and posterior leaflets.
- Without adequate room, the grippers and their frictional elements can easily be entangled with chords and interact with previously placed clips.
- When there is not adequate room, one should consider the clinical need for further therapy, taking into account the degree of residual MR, left atrial pressure hemodynamics, and difficulty of placing an additional clip.
- An alternative method is to use closure devices, such as ductal occluders and vascular plugs, to treat such residual MR.

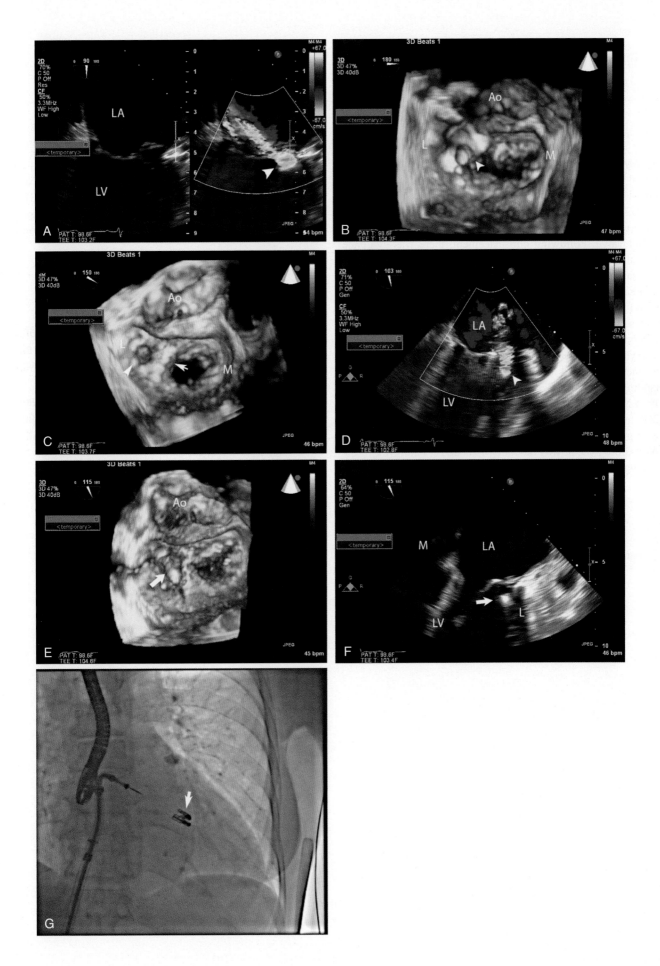

Treatment of Leaflet Perforation With Vascular Plugs

Paul Sorajja, MD

A 72-year-old man was referred for treatment of symptomatic mitral regurgitation (MR) in the setting of prior transcatheter mitral valve repair with MitraClip (Abbott Vascular, Santa Clara, CA). Three months ago, he underwent MitraClip therapy, with placement of a clip on the medial side of the mitral valve. Following clip placement, there was evidence of leaflet perforation in the A2 segment of the mitral valve.

Transesophageal echocardiography (TEE) with 3-dimensional (3-D) view of the left atrium (i.e., surgeon's view) shows the prior clip, with a perforation located laterally in the A2 segment (A, arrow). On Doppler color flow imaging, severe MR through the perforation is present (B, arrowhead). A second Mitraclip is placed lateral (C, arrow) to the perforation using standard techniques to create a landing zone. An 8.5-Fr, medium-curve Agilis catheter (St. Jude Medical, St. Paul, MN) is then used to steer a 0.035", 260 cm extra-stiff Glidewire (Terumo) across the perforation with guidance from TEE, followed by placement of a 12-mm AVP-2 plug (D, arrow; St. Jude Medical, St. Paul, MN). Following placement of the plug, there is trivial residual MR on both the left ventricular outflow tract (E) and bi-commissural (F) views on TEE. Fluoroscopic images show wiring of the defect (G), extrusion of the plug in the left ventricle (H), and final positioning of the plug between the two MitraClips (I).

Ao, Ascending aorta; LA, left atrium; LV, left ventricle.

KEY POINTS

- Devices, such as the Amplatzer vascular plugs and ductal occluders, can be used to treat discrete areas of residual regurgitation in patients with MitraClip therapy.
- In this case, a second clip was used to provide a landing zone for the AVP-2 plug, and to reduce mobility of the plug, risk of embolization, and leaflet injury.

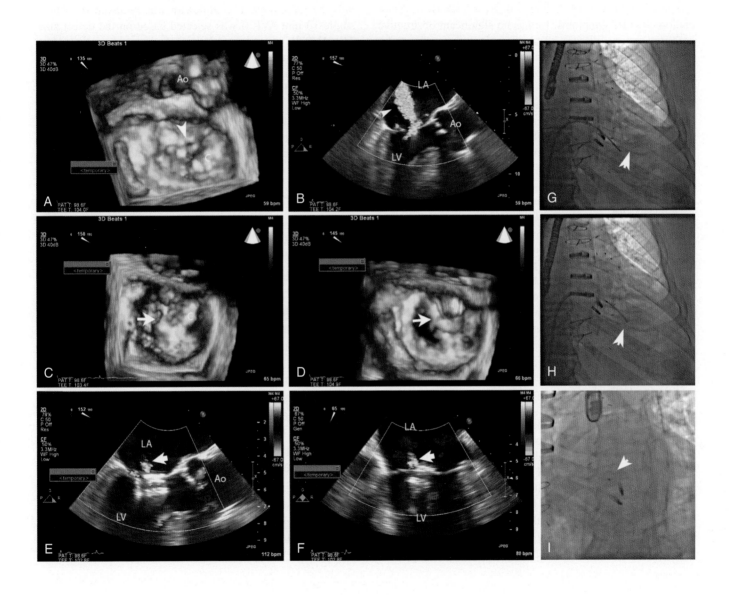

Occluder Therapy for Residual Mitral Regurgitation After Transcatheter Repair

Gagan D. Singh, MD, Thomas W. Smith, MD, and Jason H. Rogers, MD

An 88-year-old man is referred for assessment of symptomatic multi-valvular heart failure with New York Heart Association class III symptoms. He has no significant obstructive coronary artery disease. Transthoracic echocardiography confirms the presence of preserved left ventricular function with severe aortic valve stenosis (mean transaortic gradient of 42 mm Hg with an aortic valve area of 0.69 cm^2) and severe (4+) mitral insufficiency. Transesophageal echocardiography (TEE) demonstrates primary mitral regurgitation (MR) with a flail posterior leaflet (P2/P3 leaflet prolapse with chordal rupture) with an associated cleft between P2/P3 with a resultant antero-lateral jet (A, B).

The patient first underwent successful transfemoral transcatheter aortic valve replacement with a 26 mm Edwards Sapien S3 (Edwards, Irvine CA). He was seen on 30-day follow-up with persistent class III symptoms and was then referred for transcatheter mitral valve repair with the MitraClip system (Abbott, Santa Clara CA). The procedural strategy involved straddling the cleft with MitraClips on either side (first clip medial to the cleft, followed by second clip lateral to the cleft) (C). After deployment of the two clips as described, there was reduction in MR from 4+ down to 2-3+. TEE now demonstrated severe eccentric wall-hugging jet arising from the "inter-clip" space (D). TEE demonstrated inadequate posterior leaflet tissue precluding the use of an additional clip in the inter-clip space or our ability to move the clips any closer. By TEE, the residual inter-clip space measured 4.8 × 5.1 mm. At this point, the decision was made to deploy an Amplatzer vascular plug (AVP) II (St. Jude Medical, St. Paul, MN) occluder in the inter-clip space.

With the MitraClip Guide Catheter in place, we then inserted a 6-Fr sidearm sheath into the Guide hemostasis valve. We then advanced a 6-Fr, 110-cm MP guide catheter into the left atrium and, with the aid of fluoroscopy and 3-D TEE, we directed an angled glidewire through the inter-clip space into the left ventricle (LV) (F). The MP guide catheter was then carefully advanced through the inter-clip space and into the LV cavity. The glidewire was removed (G) and a single 10-mm AVP II was selected based on the defect size. The AVP II was advanced through the guide catheter and distal retention disc was then deployed (H). The system was retracted until the central waist was felt to be in appropriate position (in the middle of the inter-clip space) at which point the delivery cable was pinned, the MPA guide catheter was retracted, and the AVP II was unsheathed and fully deployed (I). Fluoroscopy and TEE demonstrated stable positioning of the AVP II and there was substantial reduction of MR down to trace with a final transmitral gradient of 2 mm Hg (E).

KEY POINTS

- Inter-clip MR can occur when approximating additional clips is not feasible due to anatomic limitations (for example, cleft, inadequate leaflet tissue to grasp). Use of an additional clip for reduction of residual MR may not be feasible when the MR is arising from inter-clip space.
- In such cases, occluder devices such as AVP II (as demonstrated in this case) or the Amplatzer Ductal Occluder II can be used to reduce inter-clip MR.
- Sizing of occluders is critical to allow adequate sealing.
- This technique works best for small inter-clip defects (~ 5 mm or less in diameter). Treating larger inter-clip defects with occluder devices carries the risk of device embolization, inadequate sealing, and hemolysis due to persistent leak.

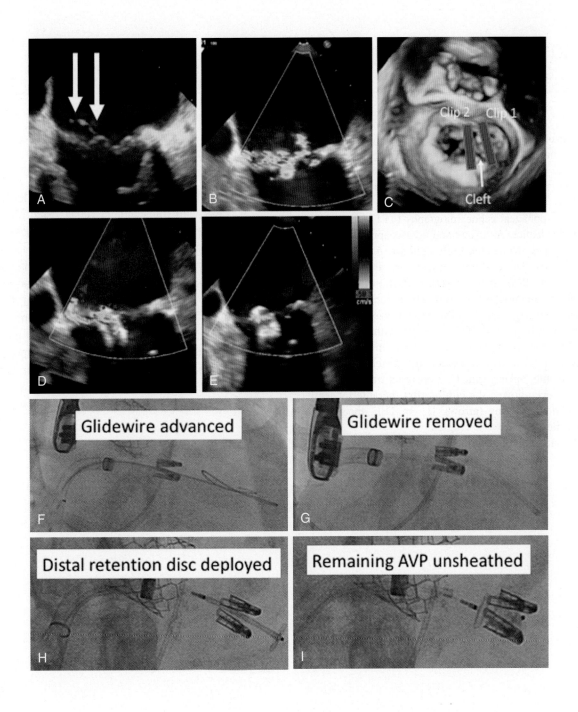

Clip-to-Annuloplasty Ring

Paul Sorajja, MD

An 86-year-old man was referred for severe mitral regurgitation (MR) that had recurred after prior cardiac surgery. One year ago, he underwent surgical mitral repair with resection and placement of a 32-mm Carpentier-Edwards Physio II annuloplasty ring.

On transesophageal echocardiography (TEE), there was a large anterior leaflet (A, arrow) and poor coaptation with the annuloplasty ring with a markedly deficient posterior leaflet (B, arrowhead). These abnormalities were associated with severe residual MR (C, arrow) between the tip of the anterior leaflet and the annuloplasty ring. D, The baseline mitral gradient was 1 mm Hg. E and F, The patient was treated using transcatheter mitral valve (MV) repair with a MitraClip (Abbott Vascular, Santa Clara, CA). The clip (arrowheads) was affixed to the anterior leaflet and the posterior portion of the surgical annuloplasty ring. G, A posterior trajectory of the steerable sleeve allowed the clip to affix the anterior leaflet to the annuloplasty ring (arrow). H, On TEE, the residual MR was mild (arrow).

Ao, Aorta; LA, left atrium; LV, left ventricle.

KEY POINTS

- Coaptation length is an important criterion for success with transcatheter repair using MitraClip. Thus, deficient posterior leaflets can pose challenges for transcatheter MV repair.
- In select cases, transcatheter MV repair can be performed. Considerations should be given to suitability of a place for anchoring of the clip, the risk of either single-leaflet device attachment or clip embolization, and choosing a transseptal puncture location to maximize the posterior trajectory of the steerable sleeve to engage the posterior annulus and deficient tissue.

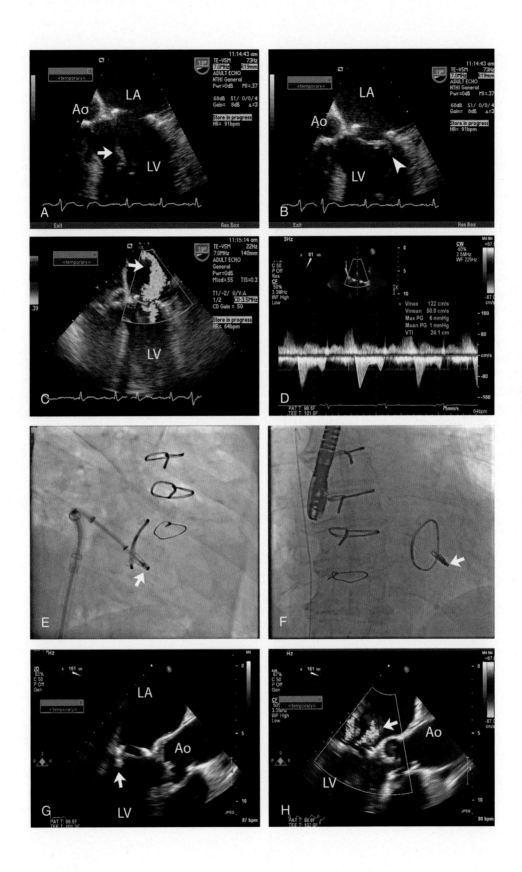

Transcatheter Repair of Severe MR After Surgical Repair

Paul Sorajja, MD

An 86-year-old woman was referred for treatment of severe symptomatic mitral regurgitation (MR) in the setting of prior surgical repair. Seven years ago, she underwent surgical mitral valve (MV) repair with resection of her posterior mitral leaflet and placement of a 32-mm Cosgrove partial annuloplasty band. She did well, but developed severe dyspnea in the past 6 months and was offered treatment with MitraClip (Abbott Vascular, Santa Clara, CA).

A, Transesophageal echocardiography (TEE) with 3-dimensional (3-D) view of the left atrium (i.e., surgeon's view) shows the surgical band (arrowheads) and preservation of the anterior leaflet. B, Severe MR is present on Doppler color flow imaging (arrowhead). C, The anterior leaflet of the A2 segment was preserved (arrowhead), but there was marked deficiency of the posterior leaflet (arrow). D, Using a posterior transseptal puncture, the trajectory of the steerable sleeve was able to be placed very posterior (arrowhead). E, The anterior leaflet is seen resting on the clip arm, while the posterior leaflet and tissue in this area are bunched (arrowheads) during traction of the steerable sleeve. F, The posterior arm of the clip is pulled against the posterior wall (PW) of the left ventricle and the annuloplasty band, followed by dropping of the arms and closure of the clip to 60 degrees. G, TEE with 3-D view showing tissue bridge created by the clip placement (asterisk). H, Final position of the deployed clip is shown. Following clip deployment, there is trivial residual MR on both the left ventricular outflow tract (I) and bi-commissural echocardiographic views (J).

A, Anterior leaflet; Ao, ascending aorta; LA, left atrium; LV, left ventricle; PW, posterior wall.

KEY POINTS

- Key factors to consider when performing transcatheter MV repair with MitraClip in patients with prior surgical repair are (a) residual leaflet tissue available for grasping, as leaflet resection is common in surgical repair; and (b) size of the MV orifice, as mitral stenosis is a contraindication to therapy.
- When posterior leaflet tissue is either deficient or absent, the transseptal puncture must be markedly posterior to ensure grasp of as much posterior tissue as possible.

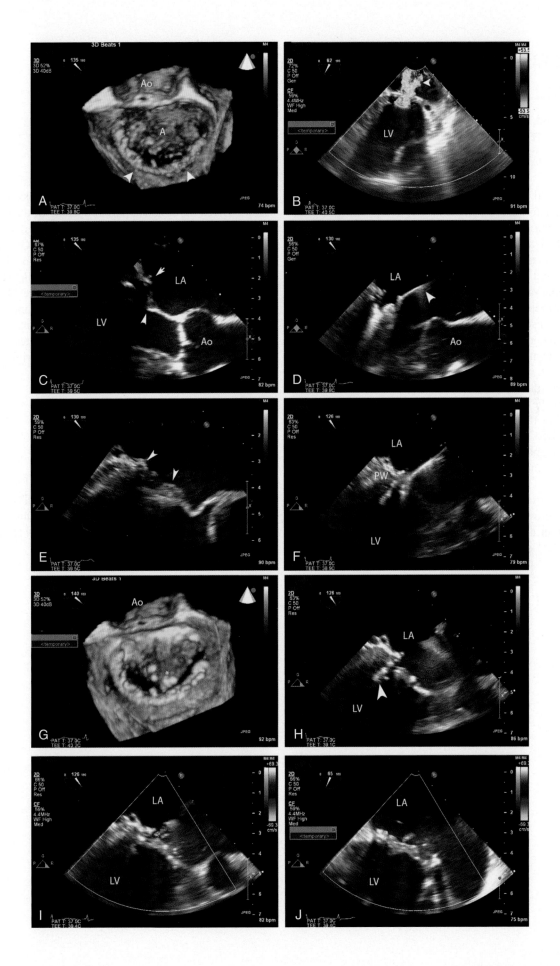

Unsuccessful Transcatheter Mitral Repair After Prior Cardiac Surgery

Paul Sorajja, MD

A 52-year-old man was referred for treatment of severe symptomatic mitral regurgitation (MR) in the setting of prior surgical repair. Two years ago, he underwent surgery with placement of a 30-mm Edwards Physio II semi-rigid ring (Edwards Lifesciences, Irvine, CA). His symptoms never improved, and he desired catheter-based repair with Mitra-Clip (Abbott Vascular, Santa Clara, CA) to try to avoid mitral valve (MV) replacement.

A, On transesophageal echocardiography (TEE), there is poor coaptation of the mitral leaflets (arrowhead). B, This lack of coaptation was associated with severe MR (arrowhead). C, TEE with 3-dimensional imaging shows the surgical ring at baseline (arrow). D, Bi-commissural view demonstrates that the MR jet (arrowhead) spans the entire coaptation plane of the MV. E, The trajectory of the clip delivery system (CDS) is too anterior (arrowheads). F, With "plus" on the steerable guide catheter and "A" on the sleeve, the CDS is realigned for a more favorable trajectory for grasping (arrows). G, A clip is successfully placed in the middle of the MV (arrow). H, Multiple views show adequate leaflet insertion (arrowheads). However, there is significant mitral stenosis with a mean gradient of 7 mm Hg (I), in addition to moderately-severe residual MR noted on left ventricular outflow tract (J, arrow) and bi-commissural (K, arrow) TEE views. Given the residual, partial opening of the clip to alleviate the stenosis was not effective. The mitral stenosis also did not permit placement of additional clips. Given that MV replacement was the only other alternative for this patient, it was elected to permanently leave the clip (L, arrow), despite the moderate stenosis and significant residual MR. In follow-up, the patient's symptoms did not improve, and he eventually underwent surgical MV replacement.

A, Anterior; Ao, ascending aorta; L, lateral; LA, left atrium; LV, left ventricle; M, medial; P, posterior.

KEY POINT

- When performing transcatheter MV repair with MitraClip in patients with prior surgical annuloplasty, the potential for worsening of mitral stenosis is a major challenge for a successful procedure.

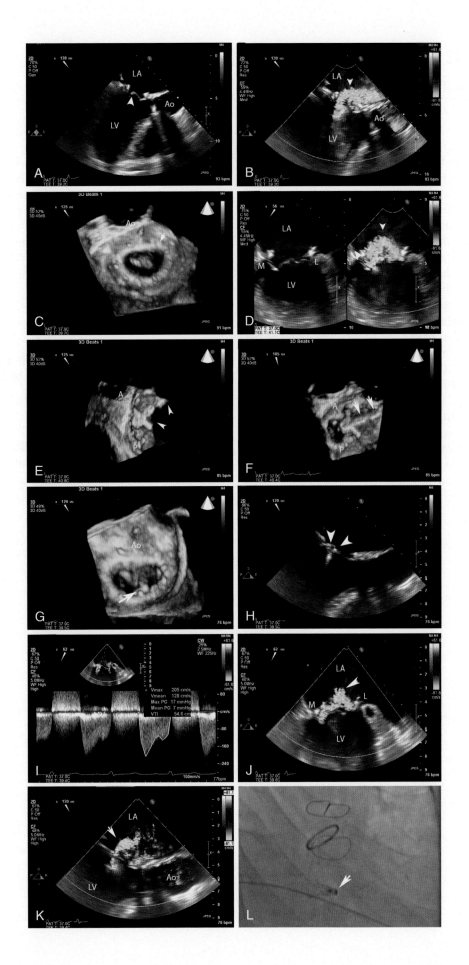

MitraClip in a Patient with Radiation Heart Disease

Wesley R. Pedersen, MD, and Stacey Tonne, BS, CVT

A 48-year-old woman was referred with severe symptoms of dyspnea (New York Heart Association class III) and severe mitral regurgitation (MR) (grade, 4+). She had a history of myasthenia gravis, sternotomy for thymoma resection, and mantle radiation last administered 20 years ago. Eight years ago, she developed mitral valve (MV) degeneration, and underwent surgical repair with mitral annuloplasty. However, 18 months ago, she had circumferential dehiscence of the ring and subsequent embolization to the abdominal aorta.

A, Transthoracic and transesophogeal echocardiography demonstrated thickening of the leaflets and apical tethering in the presence of severe MR (arrowhead). The origin of the regurgitant jet was primarily from the A2-P2 segments of the MV. B, At baseline, there was a mean pressure gradient of 4 mm Hg with an MV area of 2.68 cm^2 by planimetry. The MV annulus from the apical 4-chamber view measured to be 24 mm. C, Using a transfemoral, transeptal approach, transcatheter MV repair with MitraClip (Abbott Vascular, Santa Clara, CA) was performed on the A2-P2 segments of the MV (arrow) with excellent reduction of MR. D, However, there was severe mitral stenosis. E and F, The mean mitral gradient remained >10 mm Hg at a heart rate of 60 to 70 beats per minute, despite multiple locations of grasping (lateral, middle, and medial) and partial opening of the clip arms to 30 degrees (arrow) with moderate residual MR (arrowhead). Because of the severe resultant mitral stenosis, the procedure was aborted without clip deployment.

Ao, Ascending aorta; LA, left atrium; LV left ventricle; MV, mitral valve.

KEY POINTS

- Severe MR secondary to remote radiation therapy can be effectively reduced with MitraClip, but these patients are at significant risk for severe mitral stenosis.
- Preoperative echocardiographic parameters, including MV gradients, annular diameters, and areas, should be carefully evaluated for risk of mitral stenosis with transcatheter repair.

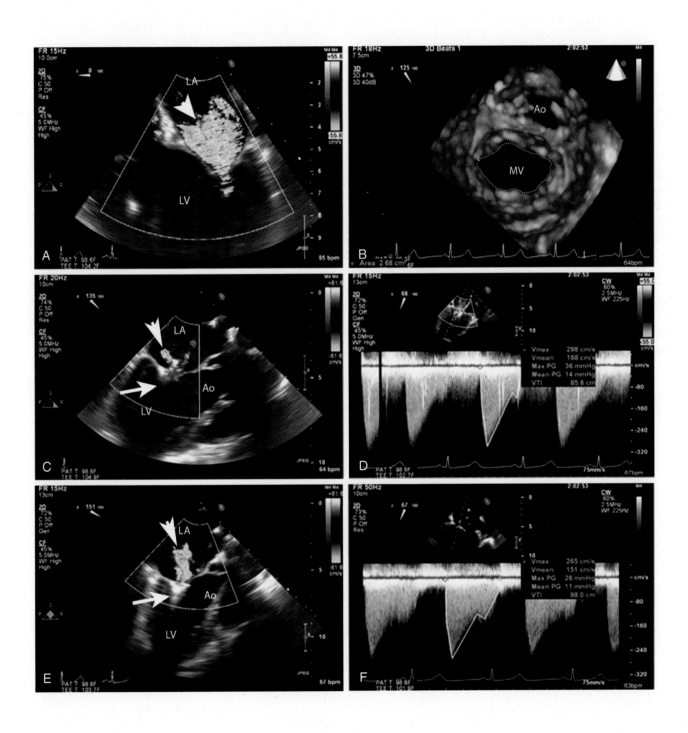

A Difficult Case of Transcatheter Mitral Valve Repair

Brandon M. Jones, MD, and Samir R. Kapadia, MD

A 91-year-old man presented with progressive dyspnea and severe, anteriorly-directed mitral regurgitation (MR) due to prolapse and flail of a large segment of the P2 scallop (A–C). He was felt to be high risk for surgery due to his age and comorbid conditions. He was brought to the hybrid room for MitraClip placement (Abbott Vascular, Santa Clara, CA). Transseptal access was obtained, and the first clip positioned with excellent bi-leaflet grasp at A2-P2 (D). Interrogation by transesophageal echocardiography at this point demonstrated residual 2–3+ MR from persistent prolapse and flail of the posterior leaflet lateral to the first clip (E, F). We therefore advanced a second clip, placing it immediately lateral to the first clip and treating the most significant flail (G). We had reduced the MR to 1–2+, but there was significant hypermobility of the second clip. The left-atrial v-wave remained significantly elevated. To stabilize the second clip and further reduce the regurgitation, a third clip was positioned lateral to the first two clips (H). The third clip stabilized the hypermobility and the MR was reduced to trivial degree, and the v-wave was significantly reduced. The final result on 3-dimensional imaging demonstrates the three adjacent clips in the area of A2-P2, and patent openings at each of the medial and lateral commissures (I). Antegrade mitral gradients were evaluated prior to the release of each clip and were not significantly elevated. The final mitral gradient was measured at 4 mm Hg (J).

KEY POINTS

- Mitral valves that demonstrate a large area of prolapse/flail often require placement of multiple clips for effective treatment.
- Despite adequate bileaflet grasp, a clip that is deployed on a large, flail leaflet can demonstrate significant hypermobility. Placing additional, adjacent clips can serve to stabilize the existing clips, and further reduce the MR.

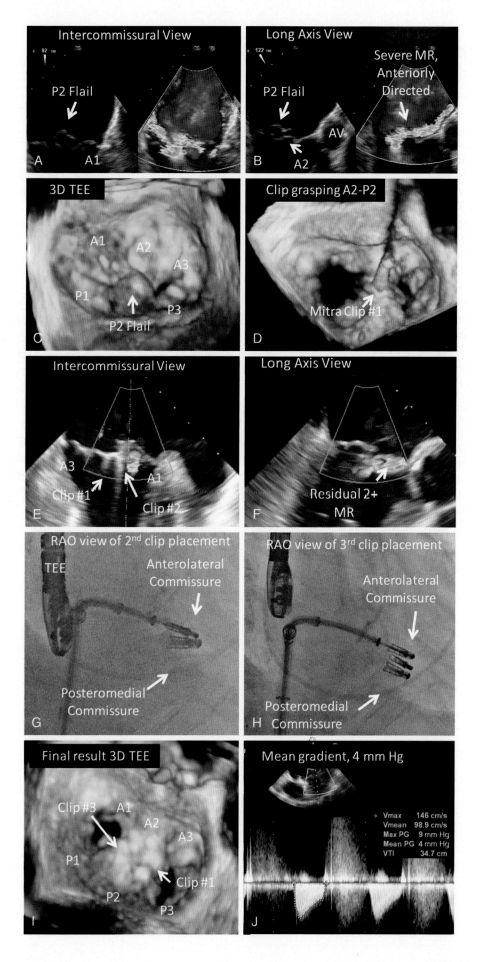

Stuck on the Atrial Septum

Paul Sorajja, MD

An 89-year-old woman with symptomatic, prohibitive risk mitral regurgitation (MR) was referred for transcatheter mitral valve (MV) repair with MitraClip (Abbott Vascular, Santa Clara, CA). Following transseptal puncture and insertion of the 24-Fr steerable guide catheter (SGC), the clip delivery system (CDS) was inserted into the patient. While attempting to straddle the CDS, it became evident that the delivery catheter (DC) handle had not been fully retracted during insertion into the guide. The lack of retraction is evident on fluoroscopy (Top), where straddle markers on the steerable sleeve (arrows) are well beneath the guide marker (arrowhead), even though the clip has been well inserted into the left atrium (LA). A, Transesophageal echocardiography (TEE) with short-axis view of the aorta shows the sleeve (arrow) across the interatrial septum (IAS). B, During an attempt to retract the clip back into the guide to enable straddling, the SGC and sleeve (arrowhead) fall into the right atrium. At this point, there is considerable difficulty advancing and retracting the CDS as the clip is positioned in the LA, while the sleeve is located in the right atrium. C, After further manipulation of the SGC, the CDS (arrow) is eventually inserted completely into the LA. D, Following clip deployment and removal of the SGC and CDS, a large iatrogenic atrial septal defect (arrowhead) is present. E, The disruption of the atrial septum is evident on TEE imaging (arrowhead). F, The atrial septal defect is then closed with a 32-mm Amplatzer ASD occluder (arrows; St. Jude Medical, St. Paul, MN).

IAS, Interatrial septum; LA, left atrium; RA, right atrium.

KEY POINTS

- For patients undergoing transcatheter MV repair with MitraClip, the DC handle must be fully retracted when inserting the CDS into the SGC to enable straddling of the steerable sleeve.
- Placement of an atrial septal occluder may not permit re-crossing of the atrial septum with the SGC, and therefore may not allow additional MitraClip therapy. Thus, in the event of injury to the atrial septum, the operator should anticipate that the atrial septal defect will need treatment, and optimize the reduction in MR with clip implantation before closure.

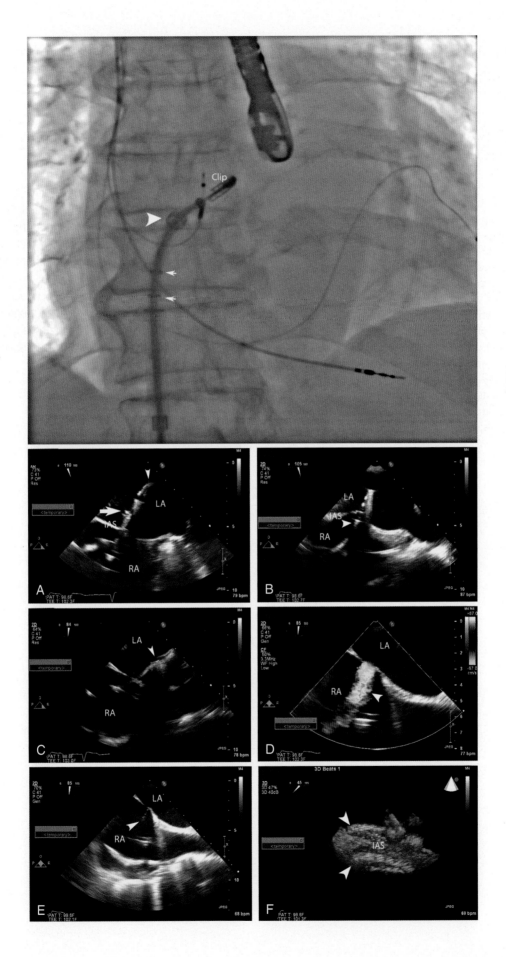

Ensuring Mitral Leaflet Insertion

Paul Sorajja, MD

For patients undergoing transcatheter mitral valve (MV) repair with MitraClip (Abbott Vascular, Santa Clara, CA), ensuring adequate insertion of both the anterior and posterior leaflets is necessary to reduce the risks of single-leaflet device attachment and of clip embolization. A, View of the MitraClip NT clip arms and grippers. The grippers have frictional elements located on the distal or ventricular side (arrowheads). The leaflets therefore must be adequately placed between these elements and the clip arms. B, Position of the grippers (arrowheads) when they have been dropped onto the clip arms. A nitinol wire loop (arrow) runs through the grippers, enabling their lowering or raising. C, Intraprocedural transesophageal echocardiography shows the grippers (arrowheads). The anterior MV leaflet also is easily seen in this view (arrow). D, When there is significant leaflet insertion, one may see the grippers rising with ventricular systole (arrowheads). This occurs from mitral leaflet tissue (arrow) pushing on the grippers and the soft nitinol wire.

LA, Left atrium; LV, left ventricle.

KEY POINTS

- Adequate mitral leaflet insertion is essential to reducing the risks of single-leaflet device attachment and of clip embolization during transcatheter MV repair with MitraClip. Visualization of the leaflets over both clip arms with comprehensive echocardiography is commonly utilized for this assessment.
- Prior to closing the clip arms, visualization of the leaflets inserting between the grippers and arms also should be sought. Lifting of the grippers during systolic motion of the MV can be useful to ensure adequacy of mitral leaflet insertion.

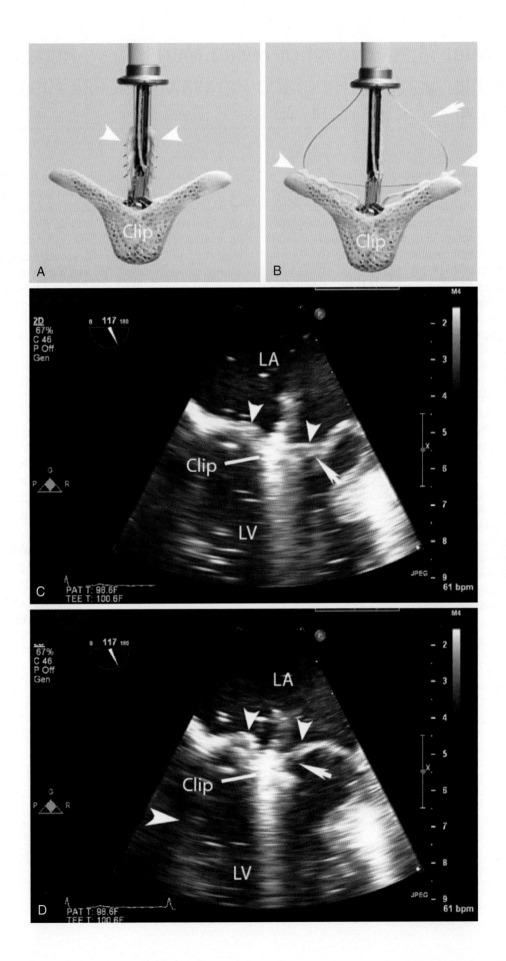

Transcatheter Management of Failed Mitral Valve Repair: Transcatheter Valve-in-Ring and Paravalvular Leak Closure

Gagan D. Singh, MD, Thomas W. Smith, MD, and Jason H. Rogers, MD

A 69-year-old woman has limiting dyspnea secondary to failed mitral valve (MV) repair. She had previously undergone MV repair with a 26-mm semi-rigid, complete Physio 1 annuloplasty ring. Transesophageal echocardiography (TEE) demonstrated severe intra-ring regurgitation (A and I) along with a transmitral gradient of 8 mm Hg (B). Due to multiple comorbidities (STS-PROM, 15%), she is referred for transcatheter mitral valve-in-ring (TMViR). A transfemoral venous–transseptal approach (TF-TS) is undertaken. TS puncture was achieved in the supero-posterior fossa ovalis. The interatrial septum is predilated using a 14-mm semi-compliant balloon. Next, a 0.035″ angled glidewire is advanced into the left ventricle (LV) and exchanged for a 0.035″ Amplatz Super Stiff Wire (7-cm floppy tip pre-shaped into a "U" curve) to form the "LV Rail" (C). Next, a 23-mm Edwards Sapien S3 valve is advanced (leading with open cells) into the right atrium. With the mitral annular ring viewed "in plane," the entire system is then advanced across the septum, into the left atrium and ultimately across the mitral annular ring (D). After appropriate alignment, positioning (middle marker of transcatheter aortic valve replacement [TAVR] balloon in center plane with annular ring), and maintaining coaxiality, the valve is deployed to nominal pressure under rapid pacing. Note the shift in annular plane (blue circles) with nominal balloon inflation (E,F). TEE assessment indicated a well-seated valve with no intravalvular regurgitation. However, there was now severe "peri-ring" regurgitation (PRR) (G [blue arrow] and I). The etiology of the PRR was felt to be dehiscence secondary to valve deployment and transient annular deformation (E,F). By TEE, the defect was measured to be 6 × 15 mm. A 14-Fr Agilis NxT sheath was advanced into the LA, and a 0.035″ angled glidewire was advanced into the LV through the peri-ring defect. Over the glidewire, a 6-Fr MP guide catheter was advanced into the LV. The process was repeated, and an additional 6-Fr MP guide catheter was advanced into the LV. Two 10-mm Amplatz Vascular Plugs II (AVP II) were prepped and via the MPA guide catheters. Both distal discs were deployed just below the ventricular side of the newly deployed Sapien valve, after which the remainder of the AVP plugs were unsheathed (H). After confirmation of secure placement and eradication of the PRR, the AVP II's were disengaged from their respective delivery cables. Final TEE imaging confirmed complete eradication of mitral regurgitation (intra- and peri-ring) (I).

LA, Left atrium; LV, left ventricle

KEY POINTS

- The TF-TS approach with an LV apical rail provides an alternative approach for TMViR procedures; this approach, by avoiding thoracic incision, has the potential to reduce overall morbidity of the procedure.
- Maintaining coaxiality during deployment is the main technical challenge with this approach.
- Deployment of a TMViR may result in substantial deformation of the natural contour of the prosthetic-annulus interface, resulting in dehiscence and resultant PRR.
- Post TMViR, PRR can be treated using vascular plugs.

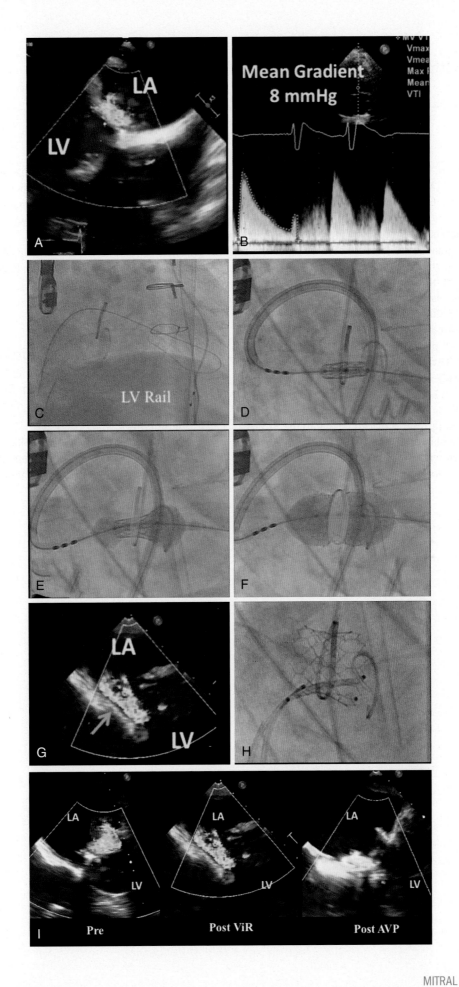

Single Leaflet Device Attachment

Paul Sorajja, MD

An 87-year-old woman, who had previously undergone transcatheter mitral valve (MV) repair with MitraClip (Abbott Vascular, Santa Clara, CA), returned for new symptoms of dyspnea.

A, Transesophageal echocardiography (TEE) demonstrates single leaflet device attachment (SLDA) of the MitraClip on the anterior leaflet of the MV (arrowhead). B, In addition, there is a flail segment of the posterior leaflet (arrowhead). C, A second clip (arrow) is positioned first lateral to the SLDA (arrowhead) using 3-dimensional (3-D) TEE imaging. D, X-plane imaging is used to examine clip positioning (arrowhead) near the prior clip (arrow) while crossing the MV into the left ventricle. E, There is visualization of the gripper and the leaflet (arrowhead), which is resting on the clip that is being deployed (arrow). F, TEE with 3-D imaging showing final positioning of the first additional clip (arrow). G, A second additional clip (arrow) is placed medial to the SLDA. H, The trajectory and placement of the second additional clip, which is medial (arrowhead), is best seen on the commissural TEE view. I, Fluoroscopy showing positioning of the second additional clip. J, Fluoroscopy showing positioning of the third additional clip. K, Visualization of both the shaft of the steerable sleeve and the clip being deployed helps to ensure that leaflet insertion is being assessed for the clip currently being deployed. L, Final TEE with 3-D imaging shows the three clips in place.

A, Anterior; Ao, ascending aorta; L, lateral; LA, left atrium; LV, left ventricle; M, medial; P, posterior.

KEY POINTS

- When SLDA occurs during MitraClip therapy, additional clips must be placed to anchor the SLDA to reduce the risk of embolization. Ideally, one clip on each side of the SLDA is placed as close as possible to reduce leaflet motion.
- Visualization of the steerable sleeve and clip being deployed in one image is essential to determining leaflet insertion when additional clips are placed.

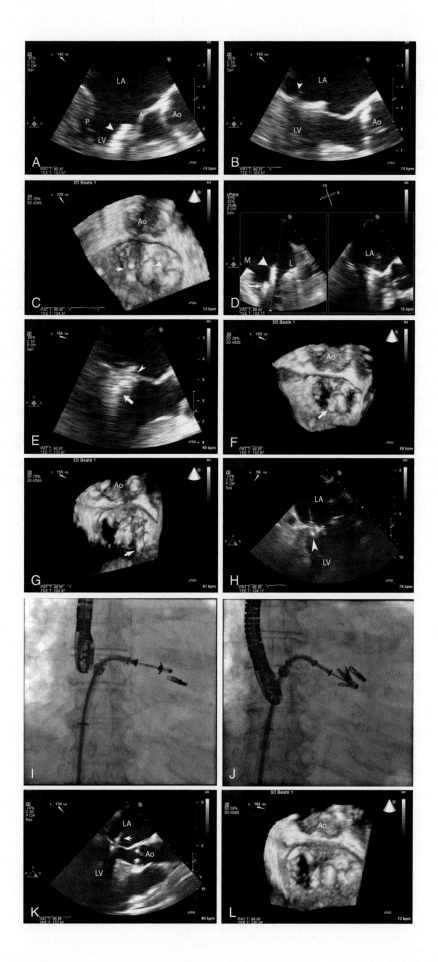

Lessons Learned From a Difficult MitraClip Case: Progression of Myxomatous Disease Following Percutaneous Mitral Valve Repair

Marc R. Katz, MD, Gorav Ailawadi, MD, and D. Scott Lim, MD

A 68-year-old Philippine woman was referred for treatment of severe mitral regurgitation (MR). Her past medical history was significant for myasthenia gravis, left pneumonectomy, a cerebrovascular accident, bilateral subdural hematomas, a left carotid artery aneurysm treated with stent and coils, and coronary artery disease treated with percutaneous intervention. Following her initial presentation, she was treated with percutaneous mitral repair utilizing four MitraClips (Abbott Vascular, Santa Clara, CA), resulting in marked improvement and 1-2+ residual MR. Eighteen months later, she returned with severe dyspnea and worsened MR. Transesophageal echocardiography demonstrated (A) a prolapsing segment, with (B) severe regurgitation next to the four previously placed MitraClips. There was progression of myxomatous disease at the lateral mitral commissure. C, The mean mitral gradient was 3.2 mm Hg. D, In a second procedure, a fifth clip was placed at the A1-P1 segments, leading to (E) trivial residual regurgitation. Following deployment of the fifth clip, the mitral gradient fell to 1 mm Hg.

KEY POINTS

- Myxomatous mitral valve (MV) disease is not static, and requires close follow-up, with counseling of patients and physicians on the possibility of recurrent or progressive disease.
- MV gradients in severe MR may be "deceptively" elevated, and not primarily due to mitral stenosis, but rather the elevated diastolic flow from the regurgitant volume.
- Commissural MV abnormalities are treatable percutaneously.
- Appropriate planning and intraoperative echocardiographic evaluation can allow for percutaneous evaluation and treatment of recurrent myxomatous changes.

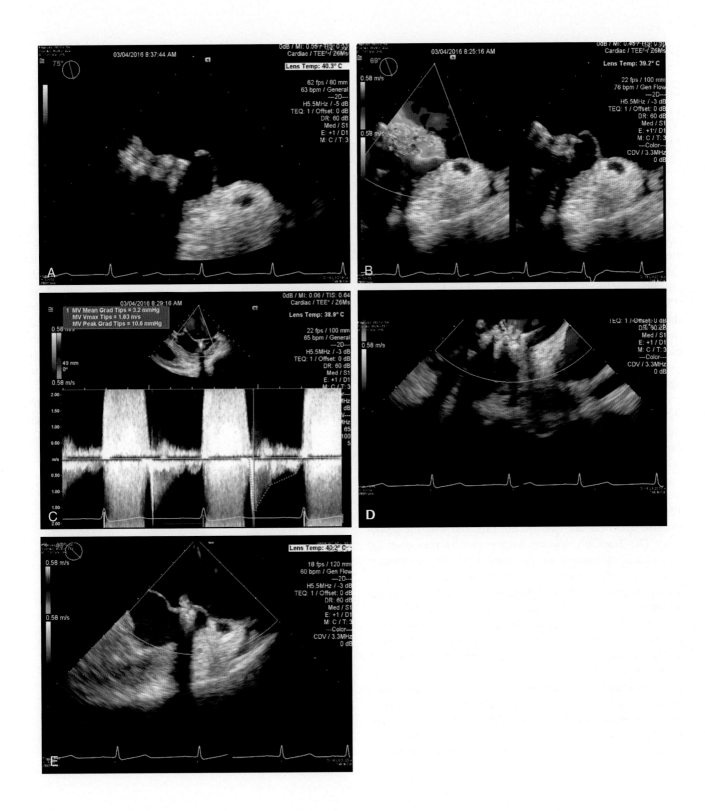

Percutaneous Treatment of Left Ventricular Dysfunction and Secondary Mitral Regurgitation (AccuCinch Ventriculoplasty System)

Christian Butter, Prof. Dr. (MD), and Michael Neuss, MD

A 78-year-old woman with a history of multiple hospitalizations for heart failure was referred for interventional treatment of moderately severe functional mitral regurgitation (MR). Due to her severely reduced left ventricular function (ejection fraction, 15%), markedly enlarged left ventricle (LV) (end-diastolic dimension, 78 mm), and co-morbidities, she was considered to be at prohibitive surgical risk. A decision was made to perform a catheter-based sub-valvular ventricular repair using the AccuCinch Ventriculoplasty System (Ancora Heart, Santa Clara, CA). A, Transthoracic echocardiography shows a dilated LV and moderately-severe, secondary MR. B, Fluoroscopy with right anterior oblique projection showing retrograde passage of the Ancora Heart guide catheter across the aortic valve retrograde, with a pre-shaped curve to access the LV below the mitral valve (MV) annulus. A NavCath catheter is then used to direct a V18 wire (Boston Scientific, Nantick, MA) behind the chordae tendineae along the sub-valvular groove and exit the aortic valve antegrade. Transesophageal echocardiography is used to verify that all chordae tendineae are free and not captured with the guidewire. The TracCath delivery system is advanced over the wire. Each radiopaque marker band represents a window that directs each anchor deployment to create an evenly spaced implant along the posterior wall, from commissure to commissure. C, Anchor no. 6 is deployed. Anchor depth is determined by a radiopaque 0.014″ guidewire deflecting at an angle of 90 to 120 degrees. Force distribution members (FDM; arrows) or spacers are placed between each anchor. D, Before cinching, all 12 anchors have been deployed into the myocardium; the anchors and spacers are loosely lined up on the ultra-high molecular weight polyethylene cable. The cinch and lock catheter is placed against the final anchor and the cinching process begins. E, The AccuCinch implant is fully cinched and locked in place. A targeted reduction of 29% (35.7 mm) of the initial length of the implant was achieved. The remaining gaps between the spacers allow movement during systole and diastole. F, Left ventriculography demonstrates a nearly parallel implantation of the anchors approximately 2 cm below the mitral ring. Angiographically, only mild regurgitation remained. G, Three months after implantation, the anchors can clearly be seen semi-circumferentially from commissure to commissure, covering 180 degrees of the posterior wall on transthoracic echocardiography (arrowhead). H, Echocardiography shows only mild residual MR at 3- month follow-up.

FDM, force distribution members; LA, left atrium; LV, left ventricle; MV, mitral valve; RA, right atrium; RV, right ventricle.

KEY POINTS

- Catheter-based reduction below the MV in patients with a dilated cardiomyopathy is a promising therapeutic approach to repair the LV and reduce secondary MR.
- Accessing the sub-valvular space and deploying intramuscular Nitinol anchors connected by a cable is challenging, but is a well-structured and defined procedure.
- Patient selection and performance by a well-trained interventional and echocardiographic imaging team is crucial to facilitate a safe and successful implantation.

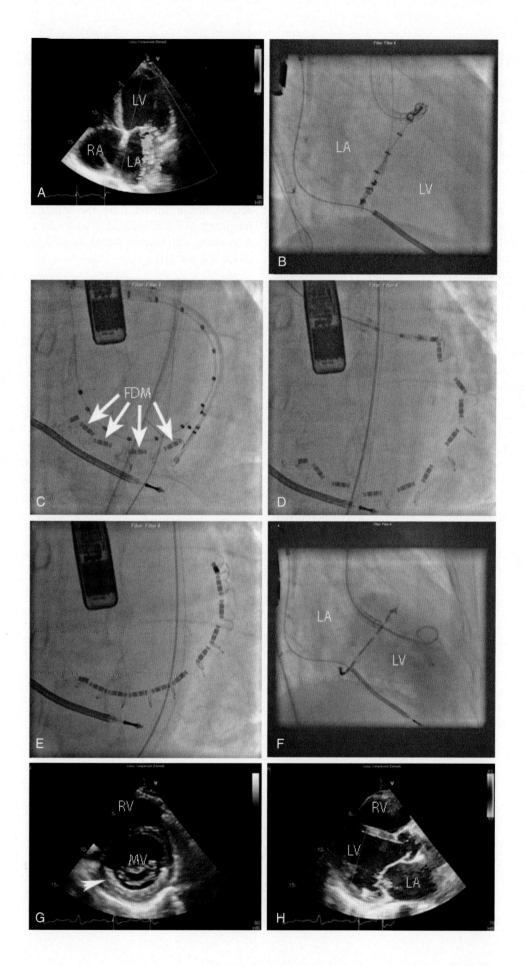

Percutaneous Annuloplasty for Severe Mitral Regurgitation with Cardioband

Shingo Kuwata, MD, Maurizio Taramasso, MD, Alberto Pozzoli, MD, Fabian Nietlispach, MD, Evelyn Regar, MD, and Francesco Maisano, MD

An 83-year-old man with symptomatic, severe functional mitral regurgitation was referred for percutaneous mitral annuloplasty. He previously underwent transcatheter repair with MitraClip (Abbott Vascular, Santa Clara, CA). A and B, The transesophageal echocardiography (TEE) revealed residual severe mitral regurgitation (MR) due to annular dilatation (A, intercommisural view; B, left ventricular outflow tract view). Our heart team evaluated him, and recommended direct annuloplasty using Cardioband system (Valtech Cardio, Or Yehuda, Israel). Cardioband was performed under general anesthesia and fluoroscopy, as well as TEE guidance. The same transseptal puncture site used for MitraClip therapy was utilized for Cardioband without the need for additional puncture. C, The Cardioband delivery system was inserted into the left atrium. D, The first anchor was implanted in the lateral commissure, with guidance from 3-dimensional TEE. E, Next, additional anchors were implanted along the posterior annulus until reaching the medial commissure. F, Using a size adjustment tool, the mitral annulus was cinched. Imaging and implantation was possible with Cardioband despite image artifact from the MitraClip. The degree of functional MR was reduced from severe to mild, with a corresponding decrease in mitral annular area from 10.8 cm^2 (G) to 6.2 cm^2 (H).

KEY POINTS

- In transcatheter mitral interventions, a staged or combined approach with Cardioband and MitraClip is feasible and may improve effectiveness of either procedure.
- Transcatheter direct annuloplasty with Cardioband should be ideally performed before leaflet therapy for MR, as this approach helps to preserve subsequent therapeutic options. However, the optimal sequence and timing of combined procedures should be the subject of further investigations.

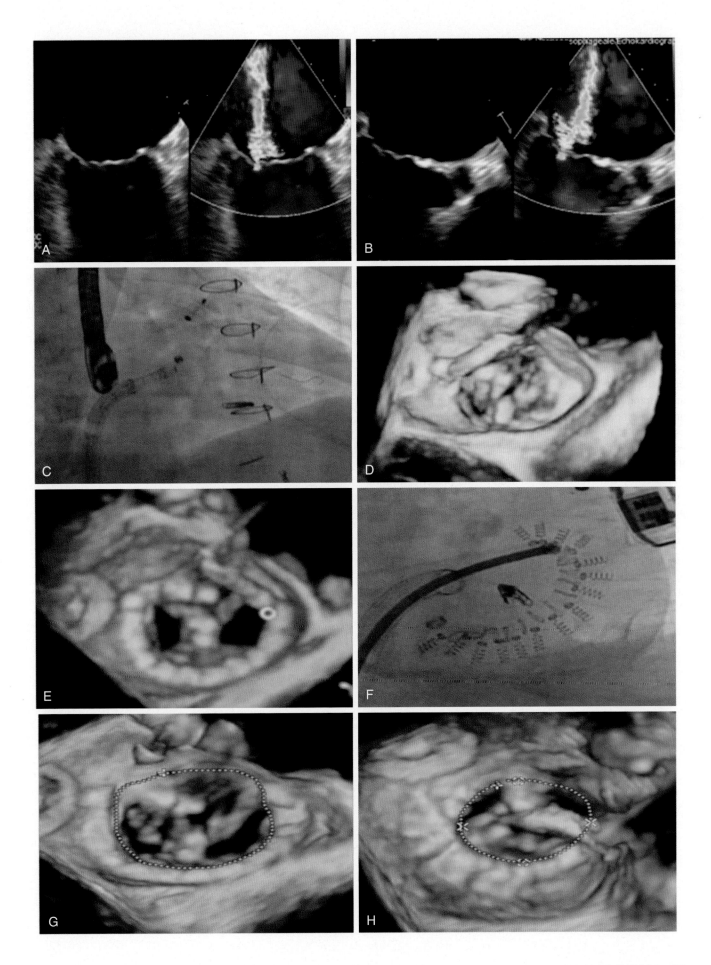

Left Ventricular Therapy for Functional MR: iCoapsys Device (Myocor)

Wesley R. Pedersen, MD, and Stacey Tonne, BS, CVT

A 74-year-old man was referred for symptomatic, severe functional mitral regurgitation (FMR). He previously suffered an inferolateral myocardial infarction 1 year ago that was complicated by mitral regurgitation (MR) and progressive left ventricular remodeling. Transthoracic echocardiography demonstrated severe left ventricular enlargement with an end-diastolic dimension of 68 mm. The left ventricular function was severely reduced with an ejection fraction of 25%. Given the ventricular etiology of this patient's MR, we elected to implant an investigational transcatheter intrapericardial left ventricle and annular reshaping therapy, the i-Coapsys device (A). The procedure is complex and carried out with guidance from fluoroscopy, including coronary angiography, and echocardiography, using both epicardial and transesophageal modalities. Pericardial space access was established with a 54-Fr sheath, through which all delivery catheters were positioned. B, Steerable catheters were positioned on the posterior and anterior epicardial surface, (C) followed by transventricular snaring of the posterior nitinol needle. The nitinol chord was established and externalized. A posterior pad with a vertically-oriented deflector was delivered on a steerable catheter and attached to the posterior epicardial surface 2 cm apical to the atrioventricular (AV). An anterior pad was delivered in a similar fashion 2 cm medial to the middle left anterior descending coronary artery. D, A sizing utensil was used to draw the epicardial pads (joined by a transventricular chord) together under echocardiography guidance, thereby reducing the MR to mild. Following apposition (E, circle; F, arrowheads), there was a 30% reduction in the antero-postero annular diameter as seen on transthoracic echocardiography (G, short-axis view, arrow; H, apical long-axis view, arrow). The chords were trimmed, and the pads fixed to the epicardial surface. At 30-day follow-up, there was residual MR grade 1-2+, and minimal symptoms (New York Heart Association class, II).

Ao, Ascending aorta; LA, left atrium; LV, left ventricle; MV, mitral valve; RV, right ventricle.

KEY POINTS

- FMR is a ventricular disease that may be ideally treated with a device targeting the dilated ventricular chambers.
- The i-Coapsys device is a transcatheter system that is sized specifically to the patient's anatomy and degree of MR.
- Reduction in mortality with the i-Coapsys device was demonstrated in the randomized surgical Restor-MV trial in this patient population.

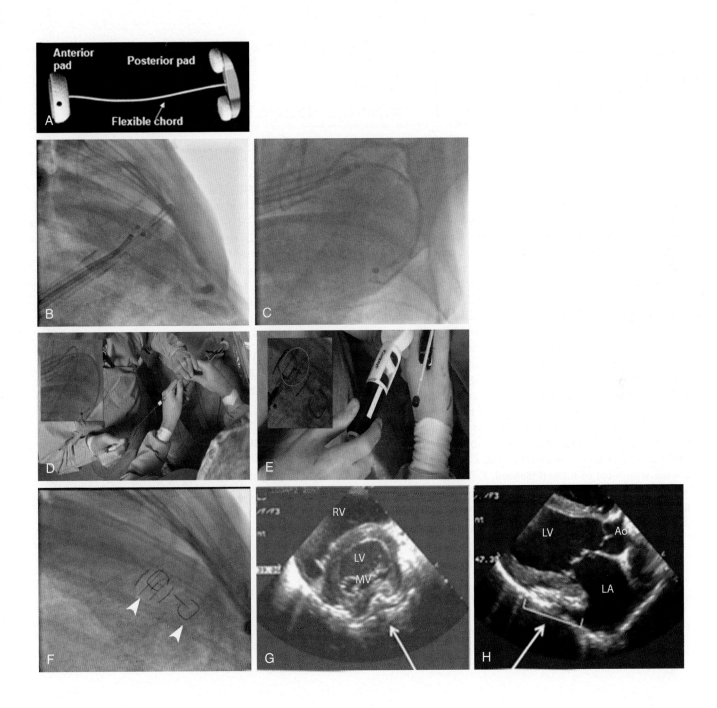

Percutaneous Mitral Valve Annuloplasty With the Carillon Device for Functional Mitral Regurgitation

Samuel E. Horr, MD, Samir R. Kapadia, MD, and Steven L. Goldberg, MD

A 61-year-old woman presents with New York Heart Association class III symptoms of dyspnea in the setting of ischemic cardiomyopathy and frequent hospitalizations for congestive heart failure decompensation, despite maximal medical therapy. B and C, The transthoracic echocardiogram demonstrated dilated left ventricle (end-diastolic dimension, 68 mm) with reduced function (ejection fraction, 26%), and severe functional mitral regurgitation (MR). She was not a candidate for surgical mitral repair or cardiac resynchronization therapy and was brought to the catheterization laboratory for implantation of a (A) Carillon Mitral Contour System (Cardiac Dimensions, Kirkland, WA). Under conscious sedation, a 9-Fr sheath was placed in the right internal jugular vein, with a 6-Fr sheath in the right femoral artery. D, Coronary angiography showed an occluded mid left circumflex artery. E, Coronary sinus venography was performed (arrowheads), and the Carillon anchors were sized 2:1 for venous dimensions. A 9-mm × 20-mm × 60-mm Carillon Device was chosen with 5 cm of tension planned. F, The left circumflex artery was unchanged after deployment (device marked by arrowheads). G, Post-procedure echocardiography showed a reduction in MR, and this improvement persisted on follow-up echocardiography performed at 12 months (residual grade, 1-2+). At 36-month follow-up, there had been no further hospitalizations for heart failure, and the patient reported NYHA class II symptoms.

LA, Left atrium; LV, left ventricle

KEY POINTS

- The Carillon Mitral Contour System is a percutaneous annuloplasty device used to treat functional MR, and can be performed using conscious sedation.
- Care must be taken to avoid interaction with the circumflex artery during deployment.
- The Carillon Mitral Contour system leads to improvement in MR, symptoms, and functional capacity.

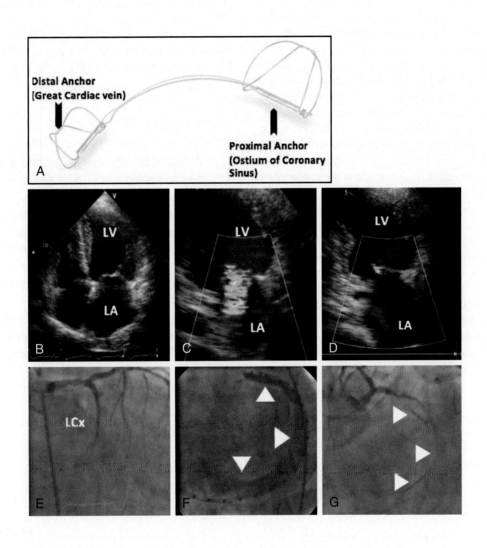

Plugging a Hole Near a Mitral Surgical Ring

Paul Sorajja, MD

A 65-year-old man was referred for treatment of exertional dyspnea in the setting of prior surgical mitral valve repair. Three years ago, he underwent surgery for degenerative mitral regurgitation (MR) with placement of a rigid annuloplasty band and resection of his posterior mitral valve leaflet. An evaluation for active endocarditis was negative.

A, Transesophageal echocardiography (TEE) with 3-dimensional imaging in the left atrial view (i.e., surgeon's view) demonstrates a large dehiscence (arrowhead) near the posteromedial mitral annulus. B, Doppler color-flow imaging shows regurgitation through the dehiscence (arrowhead). C, Following transseptal puncture, an 8.5-Fr Agilis, medium-curve catheter (SG, St. Jude Medical, St. Paul, MN) is placed with telescoping 5-Fr and 6-Fr multipurpose (MP) catheters in the left atrium (LA). The angle of the image intensifier is positioned to obtain perpendicular view of the surgical annuloplasty band (arrowheads). A 0.035″, angle-tipped exchange-length Glidewire (arrow; Terumo, Somerset, NJ) is passed into the defect and into the left ventricle (LV). D, The 6-Fr MP guide catheter is used to deliver a 12-mm, Type II Amplatzer Vascular Plug (St. Jude Medical, St. Paul, MN), which is placed by extrusion of the distal disc in the LV (arrowhead) followed by retraction and unsheathing of the plug across the defect. E, TEE with 3-dimensional imaging shows the MP delivery catheter (arrowhead) across the paravalvular defect. F, Echocardiographic view of the proximal disc of the plug on the left atrial side of the defect. G and H, Tugging on the plug (arrowheads) confirms stability, followed by decoupling from the delivery cable (arrow). I, View on TEE imaging of the final position of the deployed plug. J, Doppler color-flow imaging demonstrates elimination of the MR with plug placement.

Ao, Ascending aorta; LA, left atrium; LV, left ventricle; MP, multipurpose catheter; MV, mitral valve; Post, posterior; RA, right atrium; SG, steerable guide catheter.

KEY POINTS

- Paravalvular regurgitation involving surgical rings can be treated in a fashion similar to the treatment of prosthetic defects.
- As patients with prior surgical repair are dependent on the native leaflets for competency of the mitral valve, care must be taken to ensure there is no disruption of the native leaflets during percutaneous treatment of paravalvular leaks in those with annuloplasty bands.
- Active endocarditis must be excluded prior to percutaneous treatment of paravalvular regurgitation in patients with evidence of dehiscence.

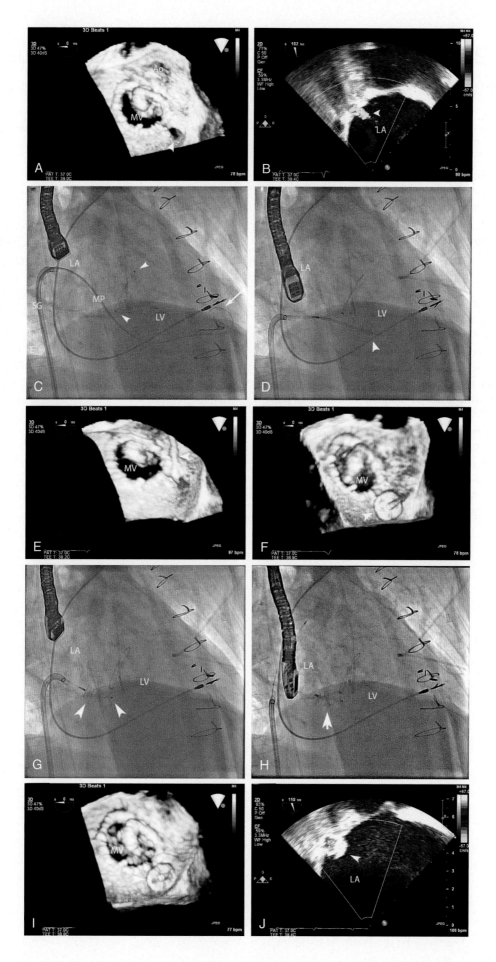

Anatomical Intelligence and Image Fusion for Image Guidance of Transcatheter Mitral Valve Repair

Alexander Haak, PhD, and John D. Carroll, MD

A 73-year-old man presented with severe, symptomatic degenerative mitral regurgitation (MR) and prohibitive surgical risk. He was brought to the cardiac catheterization laboratory for transcatheter mitral valve (MV) repair with MitraClip (Abbott Vascular, Santa Clara, CA). At the beginning of the procedure, a dynamic 3-Dimensional (3-D) heart model with automatically generated landmarks (left atrial appendage os [LAA Os], MV plane) was created with minimal user interaction based on 3-D echocardiography, and co-registered to the x-ray imaging system using EchoNavigator (Philips, Best, Netherlands.). A, The heart model established anatomical context and was used, along with overlay of 2- and 3-D echocardiography and color Doppler imaging, to predict optimal x-ray projections of anatomical features and to perform specific tasks. B, Imaging for transeptal puncture (TSP, *arrow*). C, Wire navigation to left upper pulmonary vein (PV) to avoid the LAA Os. D, Clip delivery system (CDS) navigation to plane of MV. E, Alignment of CDS to the MV leaflets. F, Alignment of the clip arms to the jet of MR. G, Localization of residual, lateral MR.

Ao, Ascending aorta; CDS, clip delivery system; LA, left atrium; LV, left ventricle; RA, right atrium; TSP, transeptal puncture.

KEY POINTS

- Patient-specific anatomy and the need to use different imaging modalities for performance of interventions are part of the learning process for structural interventions.
- Co-registration of 3-D heart models and projection onto the fluoroscopy screen enables rapid assessment of anatomical relationships, optimization of x-ray projections, and performing navigation tasks by displaying selected cavities and automatically generated landmarks.

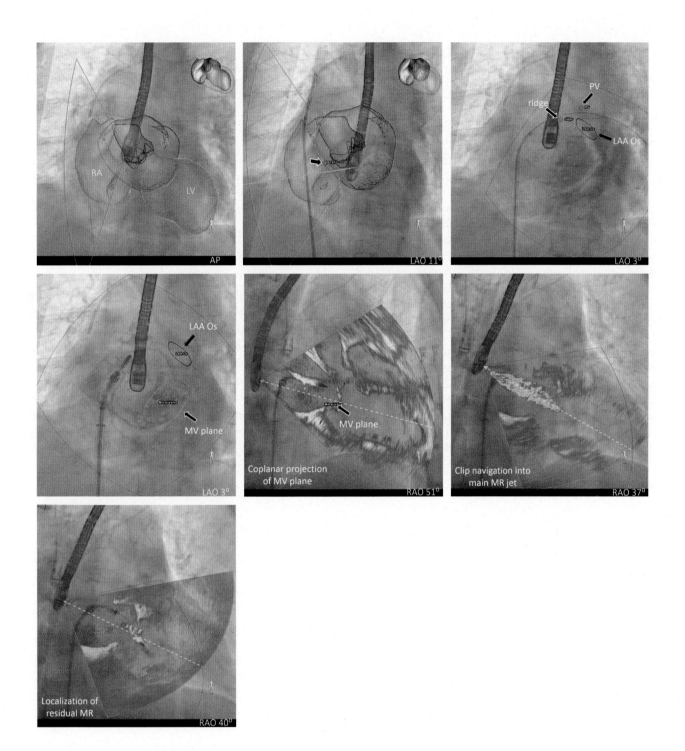

Subclinical Valve Leaflet Thrombosis

Ung Kim, MD, PhD, Shaw-Hua Kueh, MD, Mickaël Ohana, MD, and Jonathon Leipsic, MD

An 81-year-old woman was referred acutely with worsening dyspnea. Her past medical history included a prior bioprosthetic mitral valve (MV) replacement 8 years ago with a 25-mm Edwards Magna valve (Edwards, Irving, CA). Upon admission, a transthoracic echocardiogram demonstrated normal left ventricular ejection fraction of 60%, but a mean transmitral valvular pressure gradient of 12 mm Hg with an estimated area of 0.7 cm^2. Cardiac computed tomography later revealed significant leaflet calcification of the bioprosthetic MV. Due to her high mortality of repeat surgery, surgical MV replacement was deemed inappropriate and she underwent transcatheter MV-in-valve implantation with a 26-mm Sapien XT transcatheter heart valve (Edwards) via transapical route. She subsequently presented 6 months later with recurrent, worsening dyspnea. A and B, Three-dimensional volume rendering images demonstrate the 25-mm Magna bioprosthetic valve in the mitral position, and (C) and (D) ideal positioning of the 26-mm Sapien XT valve from MV-in-valve deployment. E and F, However, the transcatheter heart valve (Sapien XT) showed significant leaflet thickening, seen as low attenuation abnormalities on the valve leaflets *(red arrows)* and restricted leaflet motion. Two of the three leaflets were affected as seen on the (E) short-axis view, (F) 3-chamber view, and (G) apical 4-chamber view (G).

KEY POINTS

- Cardiac computed tomography is a helpful tool in assessing MV geometry before and after transcatheter MV replacement.
- Transcatheter MV-in-valve replacement for a failed bioprosthesis is a new treatment choice for patients deemed at excessive risk from repeat surgery.
- Subclinical valve thrombosis after transcatheter MV-in-valve procedure is not uncommon, and careful follow-up in patients post-implantation is important for early detection.

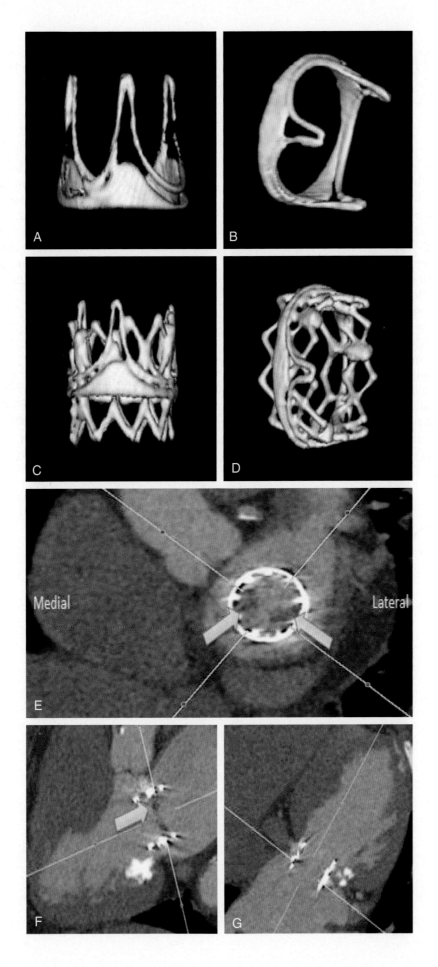

Retrograde Transcatheter Mitral Valve Replacement (Intrepid)

Robert Saeid Farivar, MD, PhD, and Paul Sorajja, MD

A 78-year-old man with severe, secondary mitral regurgitation (MR) was referred for transcatheter therapy. The patient had a history of a prior myocardial infarction and now a left ventricular ejection fraction of 33%. A, At baseline, transesophageal echocardiography (TEE) with a long-axis view demonstrates severe MR (arrow). B, Following transapical access, the Intrepid valve (B, arrowheads; C, arrows) is partially extruded in the left atrium (LA), and a landing zone is targeted on TEE. D, With rapid ventricular pacing, the prosthesis (arrow) is fully deployed within the native mitral valve (MV). The nitinol frame has a symmetrical outer fixation ring that contains variable degrees of stiffness and thereby facilitates anchoring through a cork-like effect. This outer ring also helps to accommodate the dynamic nature of the mitral annular shape. An inner circular stent houses a 27-mm valve. E, Post-implantation, TEE with Doppler color-flow imaging shows no residual MR with placement of the prosthesis (arrow). F, TEE with 3-dimensional imaging from the LA (i.e., surgeon's view) shows the prosthesis in place (MV). G, Fluoroscopic image shows placement of the prosthesis in the LA (arrowhead) with the delivery catheter straddling the MV. H, Post-implantation fluoroscopy shows the fully deployed prosthesis. I, The mean diastolic gradient across the prosthesis is only 2 mm Hg. J, Transthoracic echocardiogram with parasternal long-axis imaging performed the next day demonstrates the prosthesis (arrow) in place.

Ao, Ascending aorta; LA, left atrium; LV, left ventricle; MV, mitral valve prosthesis; RV, right ventricle.

KEY POINTS

- For patients with severe MR who may benefit from a tissue prosthesis, transcatheter MV replacement with the Intrepid prosthesis has demonstrated feasibility as an effective therapy.
- Pivotal trials of the Intrepid prosthesis are ongoing.

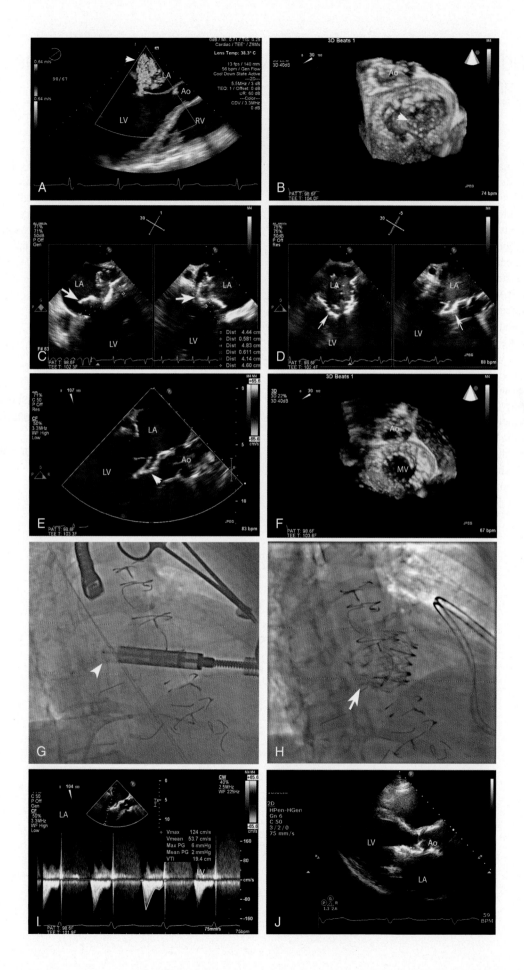

Retrograde Transcatheter Mitral Valve Replacement (Tendyne)

Paul Sorajja, MD, Wesley R. Pedersen, MD, and Robert Saeid Farivar, MD

A 75-year-old man with symptomatic, severe secondary mitral regurgitation is referred for surgical intervention. The patient had significant morbidities that portended high surgical risk, and he underwent transcatheter mitral valve (MV) replacement with the Tendyne prosthesis (Tendyne, a subsidiary of Abbott Vascular, Roseville, MN). A, Baseline transesophageal echocardiogram (TEE) with apical long-axis imaging demonstrates severe mitral regurgitation (MR) (arrow). The left ventricular ejection fraction was 35%. B, TEE with 3-dimensional (3-D) imaging from the left atrium (LA) (i.e., surgeon's view) shows the MV prior to intervention. C, Following a surgical cut-down, the operator chooses a site on the left ventricle (LV) that bisects the MV in both the commissural (left) and septal-lateral planes (right). This site is confirmed with indentation of the LV and simultaneous echocardiography (arrows). D, Using a transapical approach, the Tendyne prosthesis (arrow) is extruded slowly and then rotated to fit in the anatomic shape of the native MV. Anchoring is achieved through the use of tether connected to an epicardial pad, which also provides hemostasis. E, Following placement, Doppler color-flow imaging demonstrates no residual MR. F, TEE with 3-D imaging with a left atrial view shows the prosthesis in place. G, Preprocedural left ventriculography demonstrates severe MR, with contrast opacifying the entire LA and several of the pulmonary veins (arrow). H, Following placement of the Tendyne prosthesis (arrow), there is no residual MR on left ventriculography.

Ao, Ascending aorta; LA, left atrium; LV, left ventricle; MV, mitral valve prosthesis.

KEY POINTS

- For patients with severe MR, transcatheter MV replacement with the Tendyne prosthesis is a promising therapy.
- Studies of this prosthesis for broader commercial adoption are ongoing.

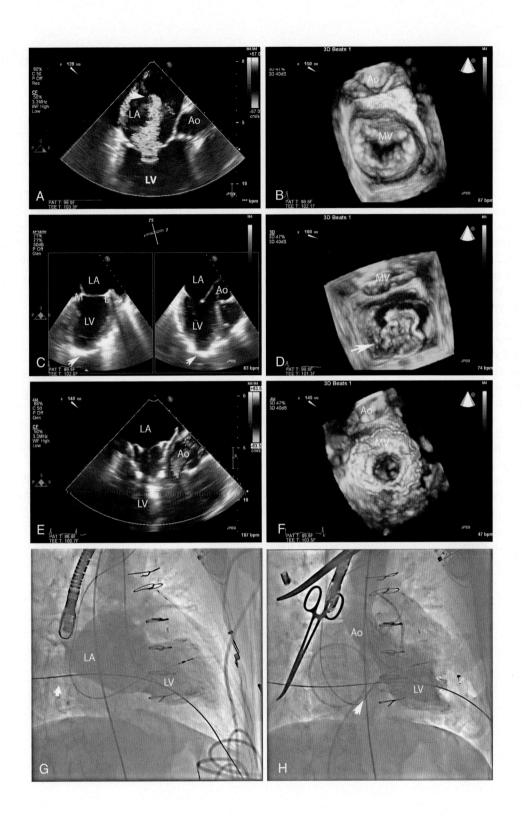

Retrograde Transcatheter Mitral Valve Replacement for Mitral Regurgitation (Tiara)

Anson Cheung, MD, and John Graydon Webb, MD

A 68-year-old woman presented with a history of rheumatic heart disease, previously treated with mechanical aortic valve replacement (AVR) in 2004, and emergent redo-AVR with an Epic porcine bioprosthesis (St. Jude Medical, St. Paul, MN) in 2013 for thrombosis. Her left ventricular function deteriorated significantly (ejection fraction, 25%) from suspected coronary embolism and severe mitral regurgitation (MR). Her symptoms and left ventricular function were refractory to cardiac resynchronization therapy, and she was not a candidate for MitraClip (Abbott Vascular, Santa Clara, CA) due to small mitral valve (MV) area and fibrotic mitral leaflets. Her Society of Thoracic Surgeon's predicted risk of mortality and EuroSCORE II were 7.7% and 17.1%, respectively. She was deemed to be a suitable candidate by the mitral heart team to undergo transcatheter MV replacement (TMVR) with a 35-mm TIARA TAMI device (Neovasc Inc., BC, Canada). A, Pre-implant cardiac computed tomography (CT) defining the mitral annular dimensions, with a virtual TIARA implant for measurement of the neo-left ventricular outflow tract (LVOT). B, Wire crossing the MV into the left atrium from the left ventricular apex. C, Centering of the delivery system using 3-D transesophageal echocardiography (TEE) guidance. D, Partially unsheathed atrial portion of the TIARA prosthesis. E, Orientation of the D-shaped TIARA to the native mitral anatomy under 3-D TEE. F, Seating of atrial skirt onto mitral annulus and deployment of ventricular anchors. G, Full deployment of the TIARA. H, Properly functioning TIARA device, and no residual MR or paravalvular leakage.

KEY POINTS

- Preoperative investigations including transthoracic echocardiography, TEE, and cardiac CT are essential for identifying candidates for TMVR.
- Transapical approach provides an easy, direct, and co-axial access to the MV for TMVR.
- In selected patients with symptomatic MR, TMVR with TIARA device provides secure fixation, excellent hemodynamics, and without LVOT obstruction or paravalvular leak.

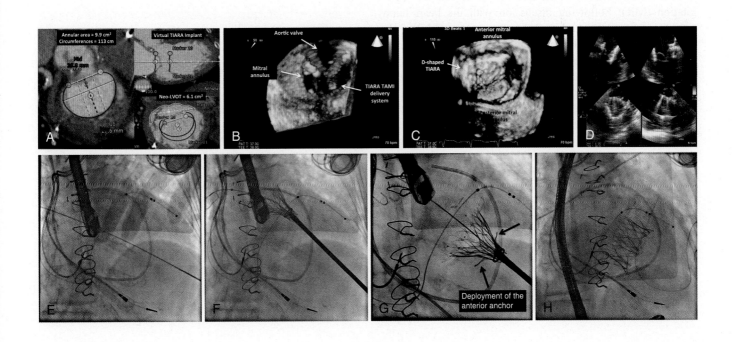

Complex Transcatheter Repair of Mitral Regurgitation Due to Postinfarction Papillary Muscle Rupture

Michael Neuss, MD, and Christian Butter, Prof. Dr. (Med)

A 51-year-old man presented with acutely decompensated heart failure as a transfer to our hospital. Four days earlier, the patient was treated with successful percutaneous coronary intervention for a subacute posterolateral myocardial infarction. Following an uneventful initial recovery, there was sudden pulmonary edema. Transthoracic echocardiography showed (A) rupture of the head of the posterior papillary muscle rupture (arrowheads) and (B) severe mitral regurgitation (MR). Following discussion with the heart team, an interventional treatment was undertaken to stabilize the patient as a potential bridge to permanent replacement. C, Using a standardized transvenous, transseptal approach, transcatheter mitral valve (MV) repair with MitraClip (Abbott Structural, Santa Clara, CA) was carried out and two clips were implanted (arrow). Visualization of grasping was challenging due to the very large gap height, and (D) immediate result showed stabilization with minimal residual regurgitation (arrow). E, After initial stabilization, the patient experienced a sudden increase in his pulmonary artery pressure (arrow). F, Repeat echocardiography demonstrated partial detachment of one of the clips (arrow) with (G) recurrence of the severe MR. The patient then underwent successful emergency MV replacement. The recovery was complicated by pneumogenic septicemia, but the patient was discharged to rehabilitative care 2 weeks after the operation.

Ao, Ascending aorta; LA, left atrium; LV, left ventricle; RA, right atrium; RV, right ventricle.

KEY POINTS

- Transcatheter MV repair can be very challenging when there is a large flail gap. In this patient, the gap was exacerbated by the mobility of the papillary muscle head.
- The weight of the papillary muscle head and residual movement may increase the risk of partial clip detachment.

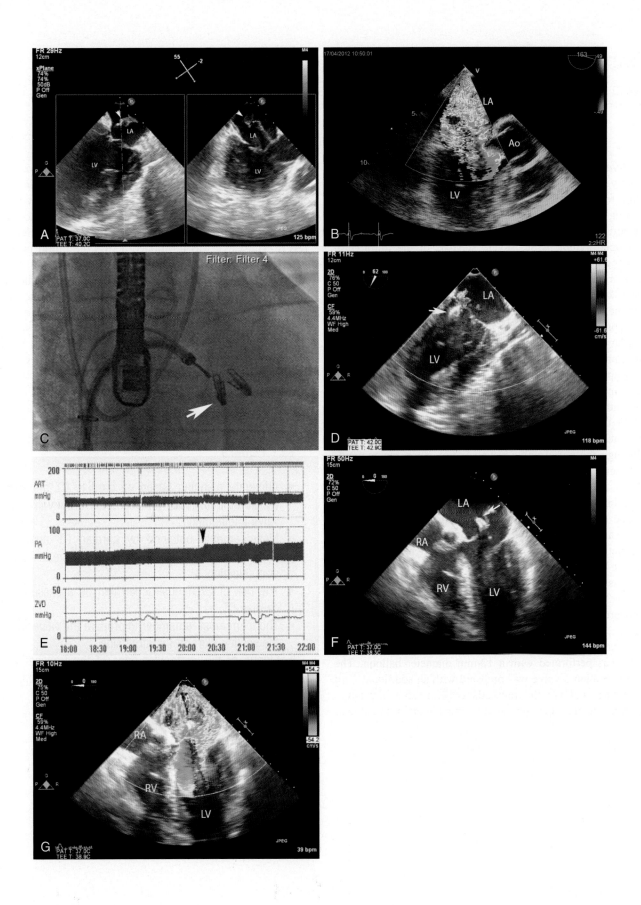

Transseptal Transcatheter Mitral Valve-in-Valve

Mayra Guerrero, MD, Michael Salinger, MD, Paul Pearson, MD, PhD, and Ted Feldman, MD

A 69-year-old woman with severe chronic obstructive pulmonary disease, 3-vessel coronary artery disease, and severe mitral regurgitation (MR) underwent coronary artery bypass grafting and mitral valve (MV) replacement with a 25-mm Edwards Perimount (Irving, CA) bioprosthetic valve. She developed symptomatic, severe stenosis of the mitral bioprosthesis (A and B). While her Society of Thoracic Surgeons mortality risk score was only 4% for MV replacement, her risk for repeat open MV replacement was considered extremely high due to the complicated postoperative course in her prior surgery, when she required 2 weeks of mechanical ventilation. She was referred for transcatheter intervention. The multidisciplinary structural heart team recommended a transseptal transcatheter mitral valve replacement (TMVR) valve-in-valve (V-in-V) under the MITRAL Trial (Mitral Implantation of TRAnscatheter vaLves, NCT 02370511). C and D, Cardiac computed tomography (CT) analysis showed an inner diameter of 23 mm, and an area of 410 mm^2. Although the mitral valve-in-valve application recommends a 26-mm Edwards Sapien 3 valve, the team decided to use a 23-mm Sapien 3 based on the measurements obtained by CT, including the use of a virtual valve to confirm adequate fit. E, The estimated neo-left ventricular outflow tract (LVOT) area was 244 mm^2, suggesting a low risk of severe LVOT obstruction. F, The fluoroscopy valve deployment angle and (G) the transseptal puncture target were determined by CT analysis. H, She underwent transseptal TMVR with a 23-mm Sapien 3 valve under general anesthesia with transesophageal echocardiography (TEE) guidance. The transseptal sheath was exchanged for an 8.5-Fr Agilis sheath and a Safari 2 wire was placed in the left ventricular apex. I, Atrial septostomy was performed with a 12-mm diameter balloon. The 23-mm Sapien 3 valve was prepared with an additional 2 ml of contrast, and with the transcatheter heart valve mounted in the opposite direction compared to transfemoral transcatheter aortic valve replacement (TAVR). In addition to correct orientation of the leaflets, this results in having the sealing skirt on the atrial side. The delivery system was advanced over the Safari wire with the Edwards logo facing down to allow flex in the opposite direction, compared with transfemoral TAVR. The valve was positioned across the mitral prosthesis and was deployed under rapid pacing at 160 bpm. J, The additional 2 mL of contrast were injected into the balloon to flare in the left ventricle. (K) TEE showed adequate valve position and function with a mean mitral gradient of only 2 mm Hg, and without MR. Cardiac CT post-TMVR showed the Sapien 3 valve in excellent position, with mild flaring of the valve frame on the left ventricular side and without evidence of migration.

KEY POINTS

- Adequate planning based on cardiac CT analysis facilitates transseptal transcatheter mitral valve-in-valve implantation.
- Measurements obtained by cardiac CT analysis should be considered for transcatheter heart valve size selection.
- The risk of LVOT obstruction can be assessed by cardiac CT.
- The team must remember to prepare the valve with the sealing skirt on the atrial side.
- Flaring of the ventricular edge of the transcatheter valve stent using additional contrast is recommended to prevent embolization.

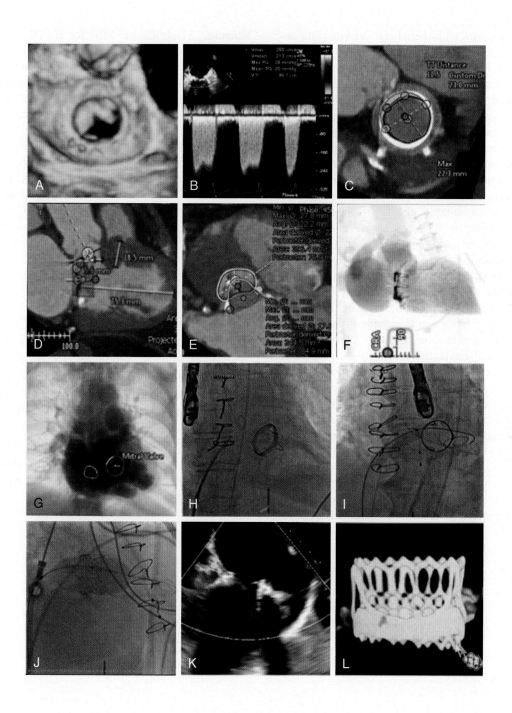

Self-Expanding Prosthesis for Severe Mitral Annular Calcification

Christopher Meduri, MD, and Vivek Rajagopal, MD

A 75-year-old woman with peripheral vascular disease, severe aortic stenosis (mean gradient, 40 mm Hg), and severe mitral annular calcification (mean gradient, 15 mm Hg) presented with acute diastolic heart failure. Cardiac catheterization revealed severe disease involving the trifurcation of the distal left main. Due to a porcelain aorta, we elected to proceed with transcatheter therapy. Following left main stenting, we performed a cardiac computed tomography (CT) scan for planning of transcatheter aortic valve replacement (TAVR) and transcatheter mitral valve replacement (TMVR). The CT scan revealed circumferential mitral annular calcification (MAC) and a suitable area for implantation (area $= 568$ mm^2; perimeter $= 87.2$ mm; average diameter $= 26.9$ mm). However, the aorto-mitral angle was 106 degrees, there was a septal hypertrophy (18 mm) and features considered to be high risk for left ventricular outflow tract (LVOT) obstruction (A–D). Thus we felt that TMVR was anatomically prohibitive. We elected to treat her aortic valve disease alone, hoping TAVR would provide sufficient symptomatic relief. One month after coronary intervention, we performed transapical implantation of a 23-mm Sapien XT valve (Edwards, Irving, CA) without complications. Despite normal TAVR function with mild paravalvular regurgitation, the patient had continued dyspnea (New York Heart Association [NYHA] functional class III). Therefore we decided to perform transcatheter mitral valve implantation in MAC. To mitigate risk of LVOT obstruction prior to TMVR, we performed prophylactic alcohol septal ablation, which has been described as a bailout for LVOT obstruction after TMVR. We obtained permission from the U.S. Food and Drug Administration for compassionate use of the Lotus valve (Boston Scientific, Maple Grove, MN) for TMVR, with the premise that a fully repositionable valve would allow precise depth of implantation, and retrieval if a significant intraprocedural LVOT obstruction occurred. Using a transapical approach, we implanted a 27-mm Lotus valve (E–H). Echocardiography revealed satisfactory positioning, with no paravalvular regurgitation. The patient was discharged on postoperative day 3 on oral anticoagulation, and returned at 1 month with her symptoms improved to NYHA functional class I. At 6-month follow-up, she remained NYHA functional class I, and the CT scan demonstrated a stable prosthesis position with normal leaflet function and no LVOT obstruction (I, J).

KEY POINTS

- Risk factors for LVOT obstruction with TMVR include a narrow aorto-mitral angle, septal hypertrophy, and a small left ventricular cavity. Determination of the neo-LVOT prior to TMVR is imperative.
- In select cases with septal hypertrophy, alcohol septal ablation prior to TMVR can mitigate risk of LVOT obstruction with TMVR.
- The Lotus valve can be delivered trans-apically, and has the advantages of repositionability and retrievability, potentially increasing the effectiveness and safety of procedure.

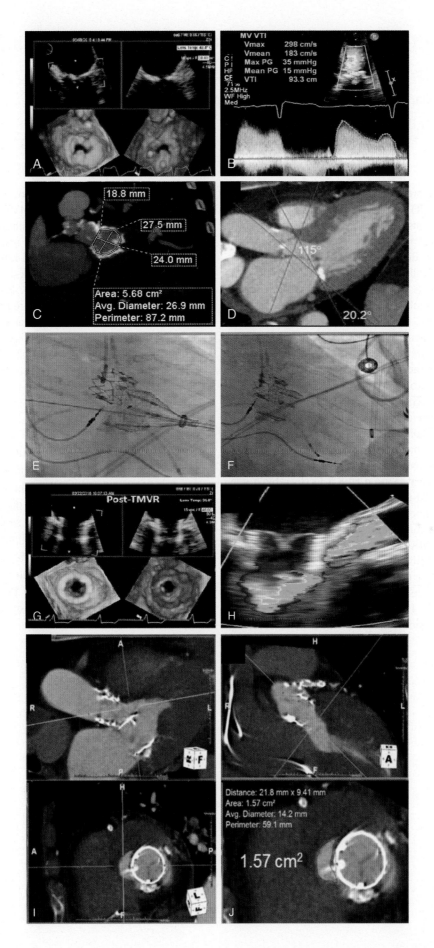

Transcatheter Mitral Valve Replacement With a Dedicated Prosthesis in Severe Mitral Annular Calcification

Paul Sorajja, MD, Mario Gössl, MD, PhD, Richard Bee, MD, Judah Askew, MD, and Robert Saeid Farivar, MD, PhD

A 75-year-old woman presented with severe, symptomatic mitral regurgitation (MR) due to severe mitral annular calcification (MAC). Patients with severe MAC are at high, if not prohibitive, surgical risk due to the potential for fatal atrioventricular groove disruption. In addition, transcatheter options are severely limited due to the risk of left ventricular outflow tract (LVOT) obstruction, embolization, and ineffective paravalvular sealing. This case was the first patient with severe MAC treated with a purpose-built, mitral prosthesis, the second-generation Tendyne mitral prosthesis (Tendyne Holdings, a subsidiary of Abbott Vascular, Santa Clara, CA). A, Transthoracic echocardiography shows severe MAC (arrowhead). B, Color-flow Doppler imaging demonstrates severe MR (arrowhead). C, Calcification of the mitral annulus and subvalvular apparatus is present (arrowheads). D, Contrast-enhanced computed tomography (CT) demonstrates a large, calcific spicule (arrowhead) near the anterior horn of the mitral valve (MV). E, A transeptal-apical rail with a 0.018 nitrex wire is created using an 8.5-Fr steerable guide catheter (SGC) and a 20-mm gooseneck snare (arrowhead). F, This rail facilitates antegrade balloon mitral valvuloplasty (arrowhead) with a 28-mm Inoue balloon, which mobilizes the anterior spicule of MAC, and expedites transapical placement of the Tendyne delivery sheath. G, A balloon catheter (arrowhead) passed over the rail confirms no entanglement with mitral cords. H, Fluoroscopy shows placement of the Tendyne prosthesis. I, Transesophageal echocardiography (TEE) with three-dimensional imaging shows the outer frame of the prosthesis (arrowheads) abutting the left atrial floor and a patent mitral valve orifice (MV). J, On TEE, no MR is evident after placement of the prosthesis. Postprocedural CT shows the prosthesis in profile (K) and en face with patency of the circular inner valve (L), and fitting of the outer frame within the extensive MAC (asterisks).

Ao, Aorta; LA, left atrium; LV, left ventricle; RA, right atrium; RV, right ventricle. Reprinted with permission from Sorajja P, et al. Severe mitral annular calcification: first experience with transcatheter therapy using a dedicated mitral prosthesis. *J Am Coll Cardiol Intv* 2017;10:1178–79.

KEY POINTS

- Patients with severe MAC are at high surgical risk and may benefit from transcatheter therapy.
- The Tendyne prosthesis has unique advantages for the treatment of these patients, including its anatomic configuration and sealing skirts (i.e., to reduce paravalvular regurgitation), the ability to retrieve and reposition (i.e., to reduce risk of LVOT obstruction), and a robust anchoring system consisting of tether connected to an epicardial pad (i.e., to reduce risk of embolization).

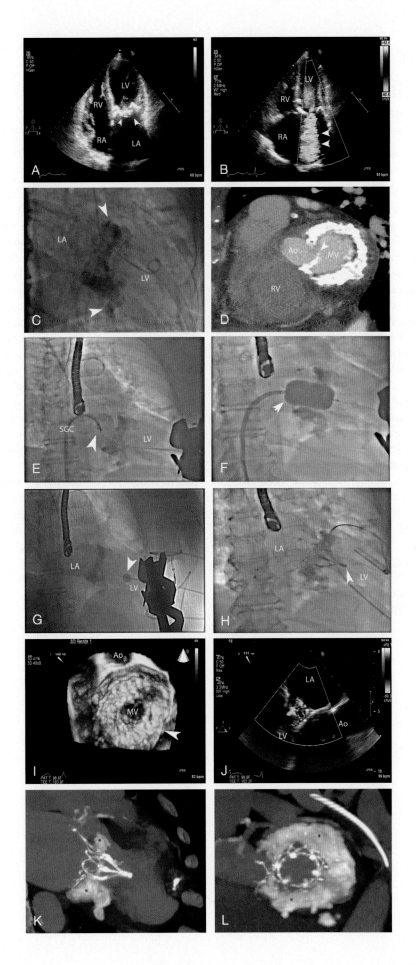

Transcatheter Aortic Valve Used for Severe Mitral Annular Calcification

Samuel Kessel, BSBME, Ivandito Kuntjoro, MD, and Gorav Ailawadi, MD

An 81-year-old female presented with "extreme fatigue" and dyspnea with minimal effort without chest pain. The patient had a history of coronary artery disease and aortic stenosis for which she underwent four-vessel coronary artery bypass grafting and aortic valve replacement 5 years prior to presentation at an outside institution. Her postoperative course was complicated by mediastinitis requiring partial sternectomy and pectoralis wound flap closure. A, Preoperative echocardiography revealed severe MS (mean gradient 14 mm Hg), severe MR and significant mitral annular calcification, with preserved LV ejection fraction. She was thought to be a poor candidate for traditional MV replacement given the severity of her MAC.

To avoid issues with her previous mediastinal wound infection and live bypass grafts, the patient underwent a right port access-thoracotomy approach with the aid of a 5-mm HD thoracoscope. The axillary artery and femoral vein were cannulated for cardiopulmonary bypass. The patient was cooled to 28°C when ventricular fibrillation occurred to allow safe opening of the atrium without entrainment of air. Although there was no evidence of prolapse, the severe circumferential MAC limited any movement of either leaflet, rendering it irreparable.

A portion of the A2 segment of the anterior leaflet was resected to minimize risk of LVOT obstruction. Although not needed in this case, a surgical septal myomectomy can be performed through this approach. The MV was then sized with a 26-mm, then 28-mm True Dilatation Balloon (Bard Peripheral Vascular, Tempe, AZ). Although a peri-balloon leak was evident with the 26-mm balloon, minimal leak was present around the 28-mm balloon. Since this patient had severe MS, this was greater comfort than could have been achieved if one of the commercially available Sapien 3 valves had been utilized. However, in cases of MAC with MR only, careful preop CT assessment is needed to ensure the valve is not too large for the largest (29 mm) S3 valve. Six pledgeted 2-0 annular sutures were placed from the atrium through the annular MAC, then passed into a 1-cm strip of felt placed circumferentially around the annulus in the landing zone. The valve was deployed under direct vision with nominal volume, leaving the proximal cuff hanging slightly in the left atrium. A small paravalvular leak was discovered, and reinflation was carried out with an additional 3 cc of saline in the Edwards balloon. B, The pledgeted sutures were then passed through the cuff of the S3 valve and tied. C, A small paravalvular leak around the P3 segment was addressed by using an additional pledgeted suture buttressing atrial tissue to the valve. D, Postoperative echocardiography revealed trace paravalvular leak, marked improvement of the gradient across the MV (4 mm Hg), as well as the absence of LVOT obstruction.

The patient recovered well and is currently living with assistance at home 1 year later.

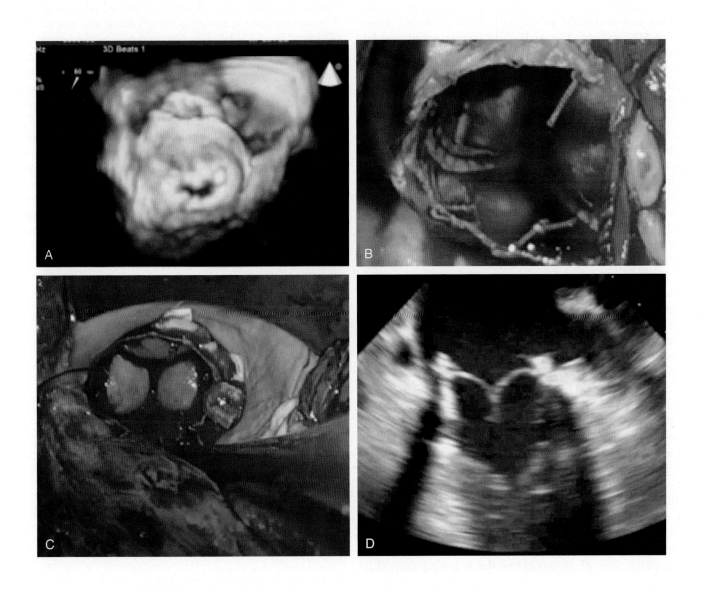

Management of Transcatheter Mitral Valve Replacement–Induced Left Ventricular Outflow Tract Obstruction

Mayra Guerrero, MD, Michael Salinger, MD, Paul Pearson, MD, and Ted Feldman, MD

A 67-year-old woman with symptomatic, severe calcific mitral stenosis (mitral valve [MV] area of 1.23 cm^2; mean trans-MV gradient, 17 mm Hg) and severe mitral annular calcification (MAC) was referred for transcatheter intervention (A–C). Despite a Society of Thoracic Surgeons mortality risk score of 4.4%, her surgical risk for standard MV replacement was considered extremely high due to multiple comorbidities (renal cancer, breast cancer, colon cancer; prior pulmonary embolism, wheelchair bound due to recent tibia fracture, severe chronic obstructive pulmonary disease on home oxygen), in addition to severe MAC. The multidisciplinary structural heart team recommended evaluation for transcatheter MV replacement (TMVR) under the MITRAL Trial (Mitral Implantation of TRAnscatheter vaLves, NCT 02370511). D and E, Cardiac computed tomography showed severe MAC involving mostly the posterior annulus and anterior leaflet. F, Mitral annular area was 520 mm^2 and the neo-left ventricular outflow tract (LVOT) area using a virtual 26-mm transcatheter heart valve (THV) was 337 mm^2, suggesting a low risk of LVOT obstruction. A transapical valve delivery approach was chosen due to a prior challenging transseptal puncture during the diagnostic evaluation. G, She underwent TMVR with a 26-mm Sapien XT valve (Edwards, Irving, CA) via transapical approach under transesophageal echocardiography (TEE) and fluoroscopic guidance. H and I, Immediately after valve deployment, there was severe LVOT obstruction with peak LVOT gradient of 120 mm Hg and hemodynamic compromise. She was stabilized with intravenous fluids and phenylephrine, without requiring mechanical support, while emergency percutaneous alcohol septal ablation was performed. J, A total of 4.5 mL of 98% dehydrated alcohol was injected into the first septal perforator branch, reducing the peak LVOT gradient to 35 mm Hg and improving systemic blood pressure. She remained hemodynamically stable overnight but developed hypotension, requiring increasing dose of phenylephrine the following day. TEE showed recurrent LVOT obstruction with a peak velocity of 5 m/sec suspected to be due to septal edema, and new multiple jets of paravalvular regurgitation thought to be secondary to increased intraventricular pressure. After careful consideration of options, the team decided to proceed with surgical intervention. K–M, She underwent explantation of the Sapien XT valve and transatrial TMVR after surgical resection of the anterior MV leaflet to prevent TMVR-induced LVOT obstruction. Due to multiple jets of paravalvular regurgitation seen with the 26-mm THV, a 29-mm Sapien 3 valve was chosen. The THV was secured with three sutures (one posterior and one in each trigone) to prevent embolization. TEE post-TMVR showed adequate MV function, without mitral regurgitation or LVOT obstruction. N–P, The mean MV gradient on echocardiography 3 weeks post-TMVR was 4.5 mm Hg, and the peak LVOT gradient was 5 mm Hg.

KEY POINTS

- Insufficient anterior calcium may lead to anterior displacement of the THV during TMVR, causing LVOT obstruction.
- The neo-LVOT area is not the only factor to consider when evaluating the risk of TMVR-induced LVOT obstruction.
- Rebound Increase in LVOT gradient may be seen within 24 hrs after alcohol septal ablation due to septal edema.
- Preemptive alcohol septal ablation performed weeks prior to TMVR may provide a more predictable response, than when performed in the emergency setting.

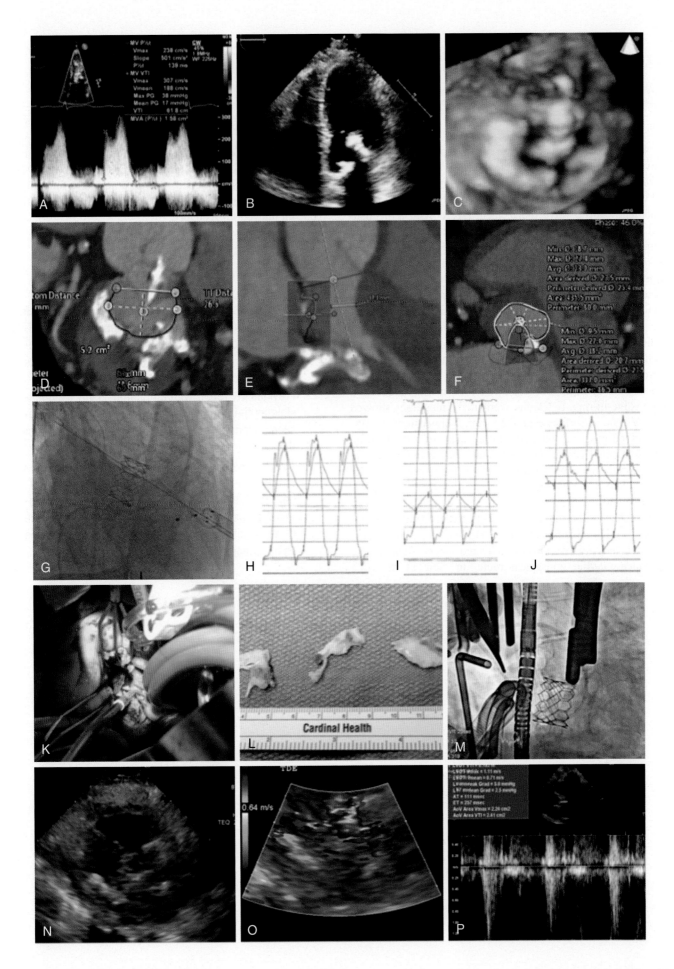

Transcatheter Valve Placement in a Mitral Ring

Joy S. Shome, MBBS, MRCP, Rizwan Attia, PhD, MRCS, and Vinayak N. Bapat, MCh, FRCS(CTh)

A 43-year-old man was referred for consideration of a valve-in-ring (VIR) transcatheter mitral valve implantation (TMVI), in view of symptomatic severe mixed mitral valve (MV) disease and previous sternotomies. He had undergone emergency aortic valve replacement (AVR) with a mechanical prosthesis, with reconstruction of the left ventricular outflow tract (LVOT) 6 years ago for infective endocarditis. Unfortunately, he had a recurrence of infective endocarditis 2 years later, and underwent repeat mechanical AVR, as well as MV repair using a 26-mm Physio ring (Edwards, Irving, CA) (A). He presented 3 years later with worsening dyspnea (New York Heart Association class III). B–D, Echocardiographic assessment showed a normally-seated, well-functioning mechanical AVR but significant mitral stenosis and mitral regurgitation. Repeat open heart surgery was considered too high risk, and hence the patient was referred for a valve-in-ring. E, Cardiac computed tomography showed an MV annulus surface area of 2.8 cm^2, 3-dimensional perimeter of 63 mm, and an aorto-mitral angle of 120 degrees. Due to a small ventricular cavity and a bulky anterior mitral leaflet, there was a possibility of left ventricular outflow tract obstruction (LVOTO). Hence, we decided to use a repositionable and retrievable device.

F–J, The patient underwent a VIR TMVI using a 25-mm LOTUS Edge (Boston Scientific, Marlborough, MA) transcatheter heart valve (THV) delivered under fluoroscopic guidance via the transapical route. In view of the high aorto-mitral angle, LVOTO assessment was done prior to release of the valve to minimize the possibility of LVOTO. K–N, Post deployment echo showed a normally functioning THV, with no residual stenosis or regurgitation. The patient made an uneventful recovery.

KEY POINTS

- TMVI is challenging given the complex geometrical structure of the MV apparatus, absence of calcification as compared to the aortic valve, and consequent lack of fluoroscopic landmarks to facilitate fluoroscopic THV delivery.
- Previous MV repair with a ring makes VIR TMVI feasible as the prosthetic valve ring provides a fluoroscopic landmark during delivery and helps anchor the THV.
- There is always a risk of LVOTO due to retention of the anterior MV leaflet impinging onto the LVOT. Careful attention needs to be paid to the aorto-mitral angle to help predict this complication. Use of a repositionable THV may help circumvent this complication.

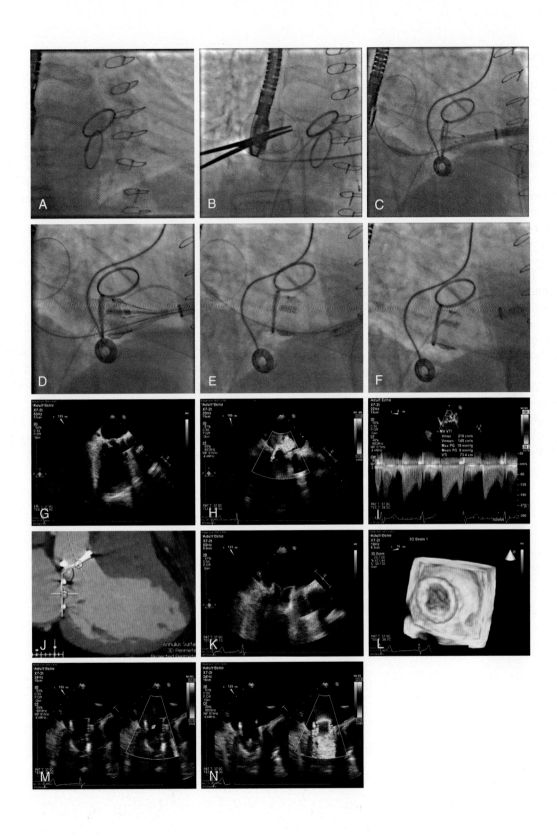

Hemodynamic Assessment of Mitral Disease

Paul Sorajja, MD

For most patients with mitral stenosis, Doppler echocardiography is highly accurate for determining the severity of the valve lesion. When an invasive hemodynamic assessment is required, the best method for measuring the mitral gradient is transseptal puncture with direct simultaneous measurement of the left ventricular (LV) and left atrial (LA) pressures. A, Simultaneous recordings of the pulmonary capillary wedge pressure (PCWP) and the LA pressure, showing that the mean values of these two pressures will be the same in the vast majority of patients. However, the PCWP is temporally delayed, as indicated by differences in the timing of the v-waves. Importantly, phase-shifting to match the v-waves is not adequate as the slope of the y-descent differs. The slope of the y-descent is damped and relatively flatter in the PCWP tracing. Taken together, the features of the PCWP recordings lead to an overestimation of the mitral gradient by 50% or more when it is used in place of the LA pressure. B, The erroneous mitral gradient (dark shade) obtained with use of the PCWP as a surrogate for the LA pressure. C, The correct mitral gradient obtained (light shade) with simultaneous measurement of the LV and LA pressures. D, Superimposition of LA, PCWP, and LV pressures to illustrate the overestimation error with use of the PCWP as an LA pressure surrogate.

LA, Left atrium; LV, left ventricle; PCWP, pulmonary capillary wedge pressure.

KEY POINTS

- For patients requiring invasive assessment of mitral stenosis, the most accurate method is transseptal puncture with direct measurement of LA and LV pressures.
- Use of the PCWP as a surrogate for LA pressure is not recommended due to dampening of the PCWP waveform and its temporary delay.

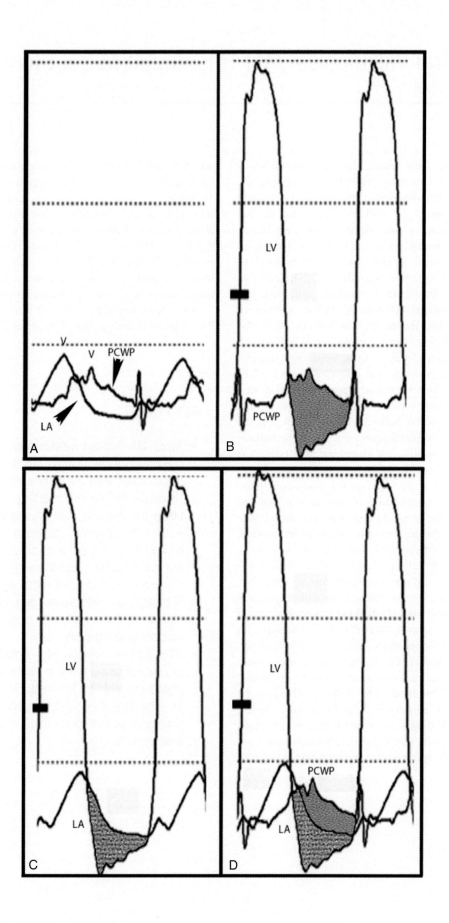

Balloon Mitral Valvuloplasty for Rheumatic Mitral Stenosis

Mario Gössl, MD, PhD

A 57-year-old woman with severe, rheumatic mitral valve (MV) stenosis was referred for balloon valvuloplasty. A, On transthoracic echocardiography, the MV had a typical "fish-mouth" appearance, the Wilkin's score was 6, and there was no significant commissural calcification (asterisks). The mean mitral gradient was 11 mm Hg, leading to a calculated MV area of 0.9 cm², which corresponded to the area measured with planimetry (red). B, On the invasive hemodynamic assessment, there was a mean mitral gradient of 13 mm Hg, a calculated MV area of 0.5 cm², and severe pulmonary hypertension. Her height was 169 cm. Using the formula for balloon sizing (size = [height in mm ÷ 10] +10), a 28-mm Inoue balloon (Toray, Tokyo, Japan) was chosen. Following transseptal puncture and dilatation with a 14-Fr dilator, the Inoue balloon is properly prepared, and placed unstretched on the Inoue wire. The stretching tube is then advanced into the inner tube, hubbed with Luer Lock, and the inner tube advanced into the W-connector. When the balloon has crossed the septum fully, the stretching tube (silver) is retracted by 2 to 3 cm, and the balloon further advanced over the Inoue wire. Then, the inner tube (gold), together with the silver stretching tube, is retracted until resistance is met and the balloon further advanced. At this time, the Inoue wire and silver stretching tube are removed and the stylet inserted. With simultaneous counter-clockwise rotation and withdrawal of the stylet, the balloon is advanced across the MV. Inflation of the balloon tip may facilitate crossing the valve. Once a balloon position without interference with the chordal apparatus has been confirmed, the balloon is partially inflated distally (C, left), withdrawn carefully until contact with the valve is made, and then fully inflated (C, right, arrow; asterisk = MV; D, arrow). Per operator preference, these maneuvers can be done under echocardiographic or fluoroscopic guidance. E, During the MV balloon valvuloplasty, the systemic pressures temporarily drop due to the complete obstruction of the MV flow. F, After two successful inflations with 27- and 28-mm balloons, the patient's medial commissure was successfully split (arrow) without significant MV regurgitation. G, Hemodynamic assessment showed a successful reduction of the transmitral gradient by up to 5 mm Hg. To remove the balloon, the stylet is withdrawn, and the Inoue wire with the silver stretching tube is reinserted. The balloon is then stretched again on the wire (within the left atrium [LA]) by using the same steps described earlier, performed in reverse order. The balloon is carefully withdrawn, followed by groin closure with either a figure-of-eight stitch, suture-mediated closure, or manual compression.

Ao, Ascending aorta; LA, left atrium; LV, left ventricle; PA, pulmonary artery; RA, right atrium.

KEY POINTS

- Avoid MV balloon valvuloplasty in patients with commissural calcification, which is more predictive of outcomes than the Wilkins score.
- Calculate the optimal starting Inoue balloon size using the formula: size = [patient's height in mm ÷ 10] + 10. Stepwise increases in balloon size can be performed if there is no significant success with the initial inflation and there are no complications (for example, significant mitral regurgitation).
- Simultaneous withdrawal and counter-clockwise motion of the stylet will most often guide the balloon across the MV.
- After balloon valvuloplasty, assess the transmitral gradient invasively (that is, Inoue balloon in LA and pigtail catheter in left ventricle). Allow sufficient time for forward flow to recover from the balloon occlusion before performing final hemodynamic assessments.

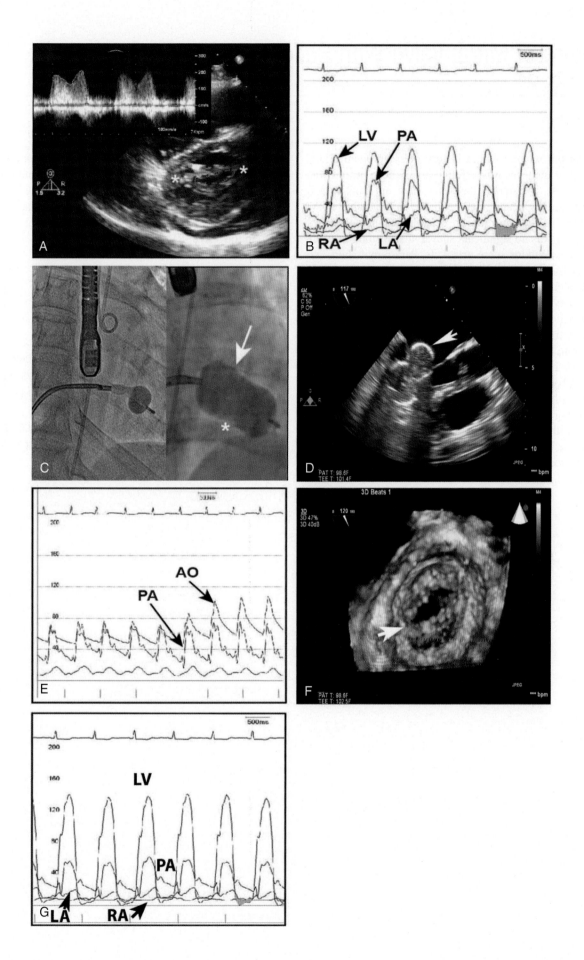

Rupture of Mitral Valve With Balloon Mitral Valvuloplasty

Paul Sorajja, MD

A 62-year-old woman with a history of symptomatic rheumatic mitral stenosis was referred for balloon mitral valvuloplasty. A, Parasternal long-axis view on transthoracic echocardiography features a rheumatic mitral valve (MV) with pliable leaflets and limited diastolic excursion (arrowhead). There was no significant subvalvular fusion nor calcification. The Wilkins score was 4. B, Parasternal short-axis view demonstrating fusion of both mitral commissures, without calcification (arrowheads). C, Transesophageal echocardiography (TEE) with 3-dimensional (3-D) imaging in a left atrial view (surgeon's view) at end-diastole prior to balloon mitral valvuloplasty. D, The mean mitral gradient was 16 mm Hg, and there was trivial mitral regurgitation (MR). The patient's height was 165 cm. An Inoue balloon catheter (Toray, Tokyo, Japan) was prepped in standard fashion, with a diameter of 25 mm. The balloon was positioned using fluoroscopic and echocardiographic guidance, with the catheter free of chordal entanglement. E, Following a single balloon inflation, disruption of the MV became evident (arrow) with excessive mobility of the anterior leaflet (arrowhead). F, Severe MR was present (arrowhead). Further

imaging with TEE using 3-D views from the left atrium (G) and left ventricle (H) demonstrated splitting of both commissures but also the anterior mitral leaflet (arrows). The patient was subsequently treated with surgical MV replacement.

Ao, Aorta; LA, left atrium; LV, left ventricle; M, medial; MV, mitral valve; RV, right ventricle.

KEY POINTS

- Case selection is key to success with balloon mitral valvuloplasty for rheumatic mitral stenosis. Favorable features include a low Wilkins score (≤8) and the absence of commissural calcification.
- Despite favorable morphologic features, complications, including MV injury, can still occur with an incidence of 3% to 5%.

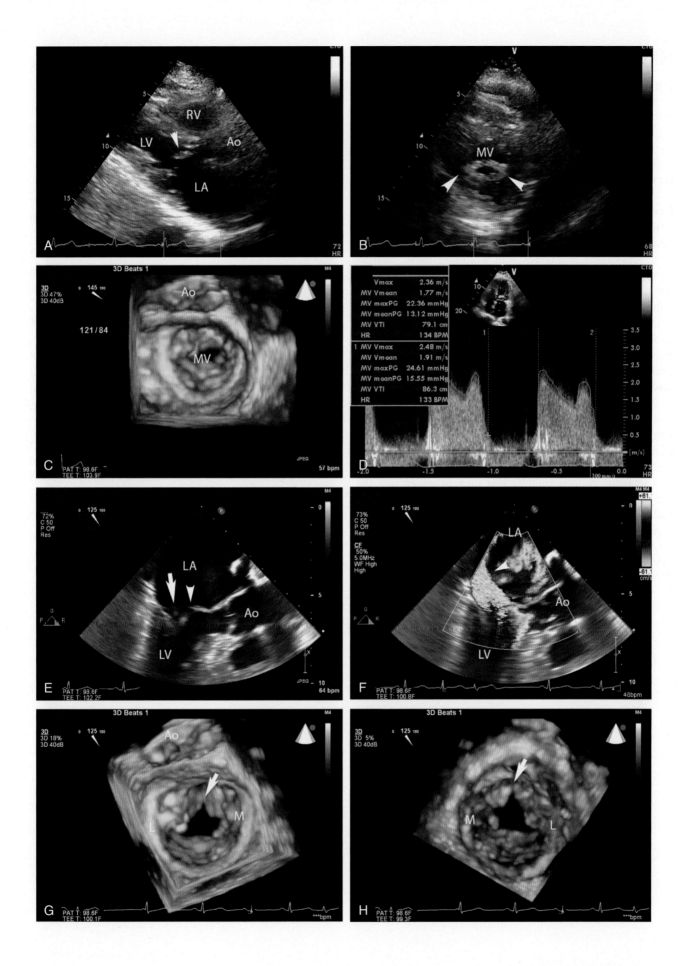

Balloon Mitral Valvuloplasty for Rheumatic Disease Using a Rail

Paul Sorajja, MD, Lynelle Schneider, MD, Richard Bae, MD, and Anil Poulose, MD

A 55-year-old woman with symptomatic, rheumatic mitral stenosis with pliable mitral leaflets was referred for balloon mitral valvuloplasty. On 3-dimensional echocardiography, there was commissural fusion without calcification (A, left atrial or surgeon's view; B, ventricular view). The planimetered mitral valve (MV) area was 0.85 cm^2 (B). Using standard, transseptal techniques with a 26-mm Inoue balloon (Toray Medical Co., Ltd, Tokyo, Japan), the MV could not be crossed. Failure to cross persisted despite a second transseptal puncture in the inferior posterior portion of the atrial septum. The Inoue catheter was then exchanged for an 8.5-Fr, medium-curve, Agilis catheter (St. Jude Medical, St. Paul, MN). C, This catheter allowed steering of an exchange-length, 0.018″ Glidewire (Terumo, Tokyo, Japan) across the MV and passage into the right subclavian artery. D, The glidewire was snared with a 20-mm gooseneck, and exteriorized through the right femoral artery. E, To facilitate entry of the Inoue balloon catheter into the right femoral vein (arrow), a 16-Fr DrySeal sheath (W. L. Gore & Associates, Inc., Medical Products Division, Flagstaff, AZ) was placed. F, The Inoue balloon catheter was then advanced into the left ventricle, with minimal tension on the glidewire. G, The balloon catheter was inflated, leading to splitting of the mitral commissures. The final mean mitral gradient was 3 mm Hg.

Ao, Ascending aorta; LA, left atrium; LV, left ventricle; MV, mitral valve; SGC, steerable guide catheter; Sh, sheath; W, wire.

KEY POINTS

- For patients with severe mitral stenosis, in whom Inoue balloon crossing cannot be performed with traditional techniques, creation of a rail using a steerable catheter in the left atrium may facilitate balloon passage.
- The Inoue balloon catheter accommodates a 0.025″ wire, which is a consideration for the creation of the rail.
- Using echocardiographic guidance, care must be undertaken to minimize risk of injury to the MV apparatus from manipulation of the rail. Minimal tension is needed for passage of the Inoue balloon catheter.
- Use of a 16-Fr sheath in the femoral vein overcomes the soft support provided from the glidewire for passage of the balloon catheter through the soft tissue in this area.

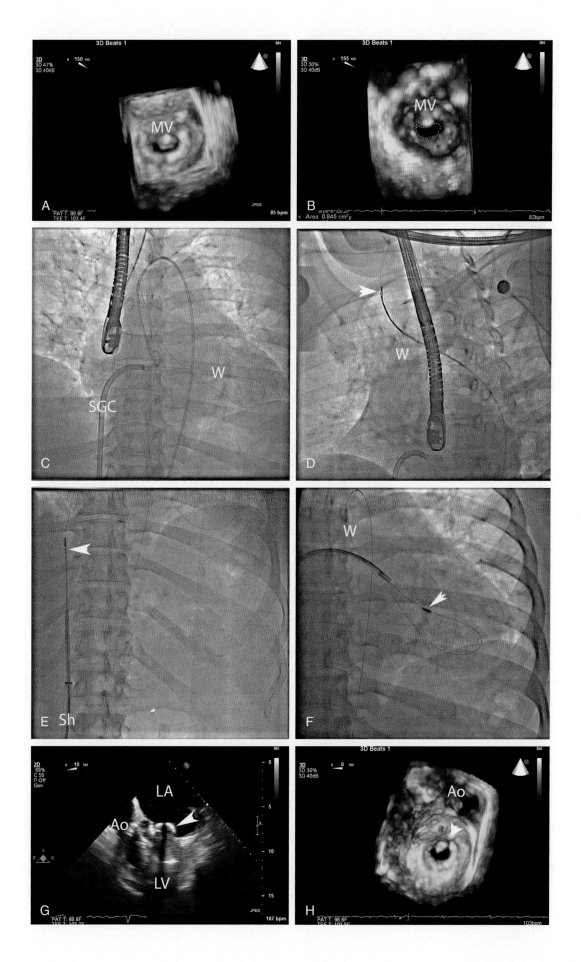

Aortic Valve Disease

Aortic Sinus Tear With Transcatheter Aortic Valve Replacement

Paul Sorajja, MD, Thomas Flavin, MD, Marcus Burns, DNP, Thomas Knickelbine, MD, and Michael Mooney, MD

A 79-year-old woman presented for transcatheter therapy for symptomatic, severe aortic stenosis. Her clinical history was significant for chronic obstructive lung disease, spinal stenosis, and chronic renal insufficiency. At baseline, the transthoracic echocardiogram showed critical, degenerative aortic stenosis (mean gradient, 66 mm Hg; aortic valve area, 0.3 cm^2), and mildly-depressed left ventricular function (ejection fraction, 45%). A, On preprocedural computed tomography (CT), the aortic valve was tri-leaflet and heavily calcified, particularly in the left coronary cusp (arrow). B, The bulky calcification involved the base of the leaflets, but spared the annulus (arrow). The aortic valve area measured 514 mm^2, and transfemoral, transcatheter aortic valve replacement (TAVR) was undertaken with a normally-prepped, 29-mm Sapien S3 prosthesis (Edwards Lifesciences, Irvine, CA). C, The calcified aortic valve was easily visible on fluoroscopy (arrow). D, Aortic valvuloplasty was performed in standard fashion with the Edwards balloon, which remained incompletely expanded at the area of the left cusp calcification (arrow). E and F, During placement of the S3 prosthesis, outward movement of the left cusp calcification was evident on fluoroscopy (E, partial expansion, arrow; F, full expansion, arrow). G, Following deployment, there was severe hypotension, and transthoracic echocardiography demonstrated pericardial tamponade (asterisk). Emergent pericardiocentesis was performed. H, Transesophageal echocardiography showed a hematoma near the left coronary cusp (arrow). The patient underwent emergency surgery, where a tear in the left coronary sinus near the left coronary artery was found. The tear was repaired, followed by surgical aortic valve replacement with a 21-mm mechanical aortic valve composite graft (St. Jude Medical, St. Paul, MN) and re-implantation of the coronary arteries. The patient recovered during an otherwise uneventful hospital stay.

Ao, Ascending aorta; AV, aortic valve; LA, left atrium; LV, left ventricle; RA, right atrium; RV, right ventricle; S, Sapien.

KEY POINTS

- For patients undergoing TAVR, injury to the aortic sinuses may occur. In this patient, the injury occurred from outward expansion of bulky calcification in the base of the aortic leaflet but spared the annulus.
- Preprocedural examination of the severity and pattern of aortic valve calcification with cardiac CT may help to identify patients at risk for aortic sinus tears with TAVR.
- Emergency surgery is highly effective in repairing tears of the aortic sinus.

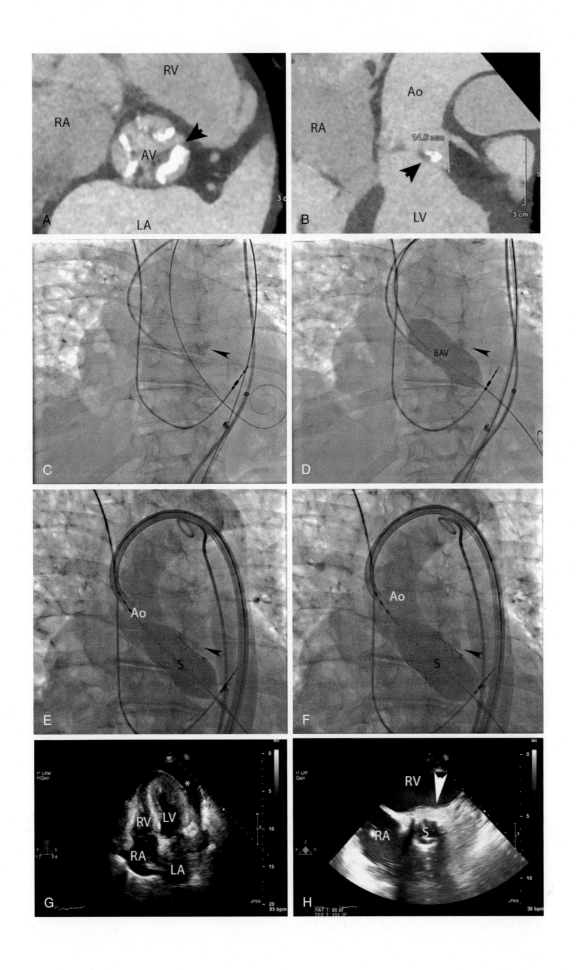

Double Valve Transcatheter Therapy for Mitral and Aortic Stenosis

Ganesh Athappan, MD, Mario Gössl, MD, Robert Saeid Farivar, MD, PhD, Richard Bae, MD, Judah Askew, MD, John R. Lesser, MD, and Paul Sorajja, MD

An 81-year-old man with severe aortic stenosis and severe mitral stenosis was referred for percutaneous transcatheter therapy. Due to his severe mitral annular calcification, he was considered to be at prohibitive surgical risk. Transthoracic echocardiography showed severe mitral annular calcification and calcific degenerative aortic stenosis (mean gradient, 35 mm Hg; aortic valve area, 0.80 cm^2). A, The mean transmitral gradient was 11 mm Hg. B, On computed tomography (CT), there was severe, nearly circumferential calcification of the mitral annulus with an area of 588 mm^2, suitable for a 29-mm Edwards S3 valve (Edwards Lifesciences, Irvine, CA). The aortic valve area measured 543 mm^2, suitable for a 26-mm S3 valve. C, With simulation of transcatheter mitral valve replacement (TMVR) on cardiac CT, the neo-left ventricular outflow tract (LVOT)was satisfactory (>150 mm^2) when there was >7 mm atrialization of the S3 valve. D, Using a transapical approach and rapid pacing, the 26-mm S3 was placed first in standard fashion (mean aortic gradient = 4 mm Hg with no paravalvular regurgitation). E, A transseptal, transapical rail (arrow) was then created with a glidewire snared by a 25-mm gooseneck and exchanged for a 0.018″ Nitrex wire (Medtronic, Galway, Ireland). F, Over the 0.018″ wire, the mitral valve (MV) was ballooned with a 29-mm Inoue balloon (Toray Group, Tokyo, Japan), followed by placement of the 28-mm S3 valve using echocardiographic and fluoroscopic guidance. G, Postimplant echocardiography showed a mean mitral gradient of 2 mm Hg with mild-moderate paravalvular regurgitation (arrow). (H) Postdilation of the MV was then performed using a 28-mm Inoue balloon, leading to successful reduction of the paravalvular leak to mild (arrow). I, Final fluoroscopic imaging of the deployed valves is shown.

Ao, Ascending aorta; LA, left atrium; LV, left ventricle; TA, transapical; TS, transseptal.

KEY POINTS

- Simultaneous transapical transcatheter aortic valve replacement and TMVR is feasible in selected patients.
- The challenges of TMVR in severe mitral annular calcification include appropriate annulus sizing, avoiding LVOT obstruction, achieving anchoring within the calcification, and minimizing paravalvular regurgitation.
- A transcatheter, transapical rail using a 0.018″ wire allows ballooning with an Inoue balloon and facilitates control of the MV deployment.

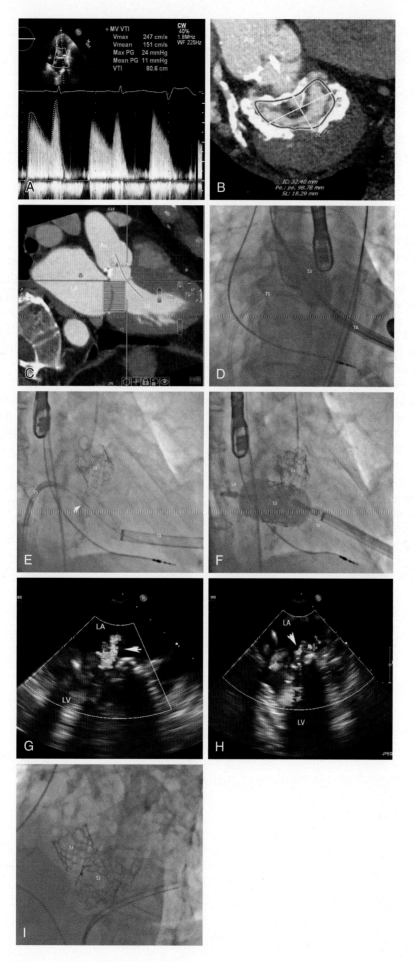

Caseous Mitral Annular Calcification Distorting the Aortic Annulus

Mickaël Ohana, MD, PhD, Cameron Hague, MD, Ung Kim, MD, PhD, Philipp Blanke, MD, PhD, and Jonathon Leipsic, MD, PhD

An 85-year-old man with severe aortic stenosis is being considered for transcatheter aortic valve replacement (TAVR).

The patient subsequently underwent cardiac computed tomography angiography (CTA) with ECG synchronization and full cardiac cycle acquisition. The coronal oblique view displayed a hyperdense lesion, with smooth margins, measuring 21 × 18 × 13 mm, situated below and abutting the left coronary cusp (A), with a partially calcified rim. The mass resulted in distortion and deformation of the aortic annulus, giving a D-shaped appearance (B, dotted line). This lesion did not undergo dynamic change throughout the cardiac cycle, with the left coronary artery lying near the lesion (B, arrows). A coronal maximum intensity projection (C) and 3-dimensional volume rendered reconstruction (D) confirmed that the lesion is in direct continuity with extensive mitral annular calcifications (MACs). This imaging helped to establish a final diagnosis of caseous MAC extending along the intervalvular fibrosa to the subannular aorta, and resulting in compression of the aortic annulus. After discussion in multidisciplinary heart team rounds, the patient was declined for TAVR, owing to concerns regarding an increased risk of significant paravalvular regurgitation.

Ao, Ascending aorta; LA, left artery; LV, left ventricle; RA, right artery; RV, right ventricle.

KEY POINTS

- In addition to accurate measurements of the aortic annulus, cardiac CTA provides important anatomical detail of the root and left ventricular outflow tract. Adverse root features such as extensive subannular calcifications, low coronary ostial height, and shallow sinus of Valsalva must be taken into account.
- The differential diagnosis for a hyperdense lesion below an aortic cusp includes pseudoaneurysm (congenital or secondary to infective endocarditis), coronary artery aneurysm, and caseous MAC.
- MAC can masquerade as a contrast-filled aneurysm owing to the liquefied nature of the calcification, particularly when in uncommon locations, as with this case. When the diagnosis is challenging, a noncontrast computed tomography acquisition can be extremely helpful to delineate the calcific nature of MAC.

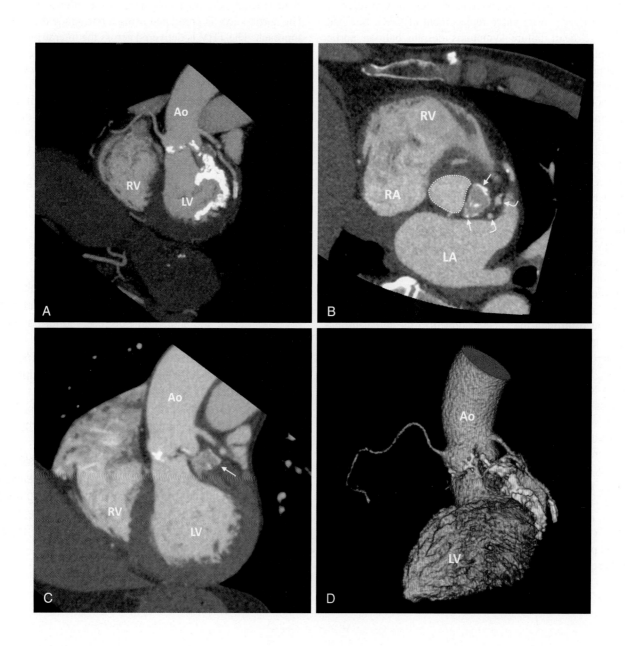

Transvenous Antegrade Transcatheter Aortic Valve Replacement

Mauricio G. Cohen, MD, FACC, FSCAI

A 78-year-old woman with severe aortic stenosis was referred for transcatheter aortic valve replacement (TAVR). She had progressive heart failure symptoms despite balloon aortic valvuloplasty performed 3 months prior to presentation. She was inoperable (Society of Thoracic Surgeons Predicted Risk of Mortality, 9.9%) with severe morbidities, including porcelain aorta, severe chronic obstructive pulmonary disease, peripheral vascular disease with previous femoral-popliteal bypass grafting, and carotid stenting. Therefore she was not suitable for transfemoral, transapical, or direct aortic access for TAVR. A transvenous transseptal antegrade approach was considered.

A, A balloon-expandable transcatheter heart valve (THV) (Edwards Lifesciences, Irvine, CA), sized according to the aortic annulus, is mounted on a valvuloplasty balloon with the THV skirt oriented proximally in the balloon for antegrade delivery. B, Transseptal puncture is performed under transesophageal echocardiography guidance aiming toward the posterior-superior portion of the fossa ovale using a Mullins or SL1 sheath. C, A 7-Fr balloon-tipped catheter is advanced through the sheath, looped in the left ventricle (LV) to guide the passage of a 0.035″ floppy-tipped Wholey wire across the aortic valve into the ascending aorta and arch. D, The balloon-tipped catheter is exchanged for a 6-Fr, 125-cm-long multipurpose catheter. The catheter tip is placed as far as possible in the descending aorta and the Wholey wire is swapped for a 400-cm, flexible shaft 0.035″ nitinol wire (Nitrex, EV3, Medtronic, Dublin, Ireland), which is then snared using a 12- to 20-mm, three-lobed vascular snare (Atrieve, Angiotech, Vancouver, Canada), and externalized through the left femoral artery. E, A 6-Fr MPA1 guiding catheter is advanced retrograde over the externalized wire into the aortic root to maintain control of the wire loop in the LV. The transseptal sheath is removed, and atrial septostomy is performed using a 14 × 50-mm esophageal balloon. F, Subsequently, an Edwards eSheath is placed in the femoral

vein, reaching the upper segment of the inferior vena cava. The aortic valve is predilated using a retrograde or antegrade approach. The THV is delivered across the interatrial septum, through the mitral valve (MV), looping in the LV, and positioned across the aortic valve. G and H, The retrograde multipurpose guiding catheter is positioned against the tip of the antegrade delivery balloon to prevent upward displacement of the valve during deployment. The THV is then deployed under rapid right ventricular pacing. After implantation, the guidewire is withdrawn through a catheter to protect the MV and interatrial septum from guidewire laceration. Venous hemostasis can be achieved using pre-closure, a figure-of-8 stitch, or manual pressure.

KEY POINTS

- Transseptal antegrade TAVR is a complex multistep procedure that requires careful planning, multiple operators, and should only be reserved for patients without other vascular access.
- Posterior-superior transseptal puncture is important to allow catheter navigation in the left atrium to create the left ventricular loop.
- Use of a flexible nitinol wire that does not kink is crucial for advancement of the THV through the left ventricular loop.
- Impingement and injury of the MV are risks of these procedures. Avoid putting too much tension and straightening of the left ventricular loop wire by applying gentle pressure from each wire end. Always remove the wire using catheters to avoid laceration of the MV.

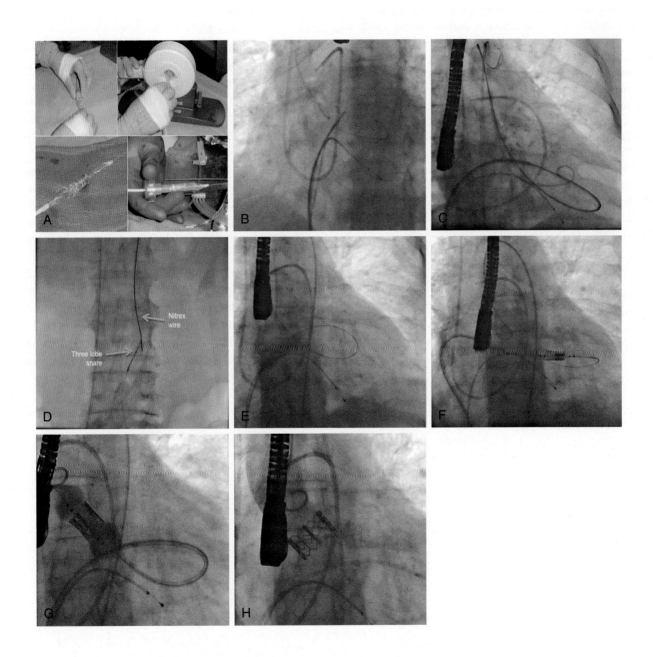

Valve Embolization in Transcatheter Aortic Valve Replacement

Paul Sorajja, MD

An 83-year-old woman with inoperable, severe aortic stenosis, presented for transcatheter aortic valve replacement. Echocardiography demonstrates a calcific aortic valve on short-axis imaging and mild hypertrophy of the ventricular septum on long-axis imaging. There is a severe stenosis with a mean gradient of 62 mm Hg. A, A 26-mm Sapien balloon expandable prosthesis (S) is placed from the right transfemoral artery. Note the position of the prosthesis (arrow) relative to the aortic root (arrowheads). B, When the pigtail catheter is pulled during valve deployment, the temporary pacemaker (TMP) is also moved and there is loss of ventricular capture. C, The expanded valve embolizes to the ascending aorta. D, The deployment balloon is reinflated to hold the prosthesis, which is then pulled gently into the descending aorta (arrowhead), where it is fully deployed. Echocardiography shows the prosthesis to be functioning normally in the descending aorta. E, A second prosthesis is advanced and positioned lower (arrowhead) relative to the aortic root with complete pacemaker capture (note curvature of TPM). F, Final fluoroscopy shows the first (arrowhead) and second (arrow) prostheses.

Ao, Ascending aorta; AV, aortic valve; S, Sapien prosthesis; TPM, temporary pacemaker.

KEY POINTS

- Valve embolization may occur due to loss of ventricular standstill during deployment, a deployment position that is too high or too low, or inadequate size of the prosthesis. While no valve embolization is desired, embolization into the aorta is easier to manage than loss of the prosthesis into the left ventricle.
- The most important step in management of valve embolization is maintenance of the guidewire through the valve to maintain the valve orientation and antegrade flow. Balloon capture and repositioning can then be performed with the guidewire in place.
- Placement of the embolized prosthesis in the descending aorta where the aortic diameter matches the prosthesis size helps to reduce the risk of further migration. This diameter should be obtained from the preprocedural computed tomography scan, and full apposition should be confirmed with either echocardiography or angiography.

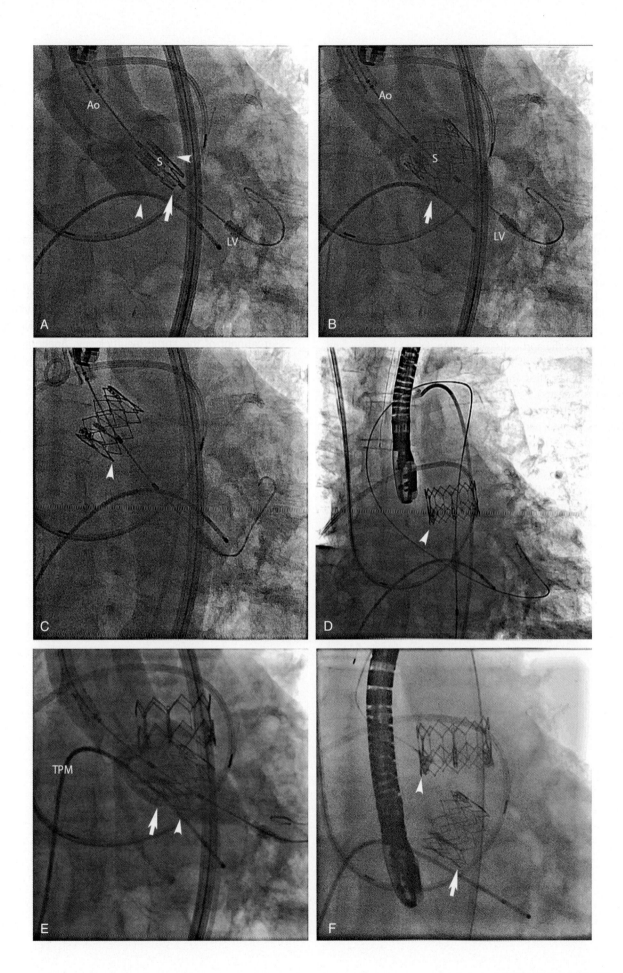

Transcatheter Aortic Valve Therapy for Ascending Aortic Dissection

Paul Sorajja, MD

A 68-year-old man was transferred for acute management of aortic regurgitation in the setting of recent aortic surgery. One month ago, he underwent repair of a type A ascending aortic dissection with placement of a 32-mm Terumo Gel-weave interposition graft. The procedure was complicated by encephalopathy, renal artery dissection, and left leg ischemia requiring a fasciotomy. He was found to have a new aortic dissection flap with severe aortic regurgitation, and was referred for transcatheter therapy due to his multiple morbidities. Preprocedural imaging with transesophageal echocardiography shows the aortic dissection flap on (A) long-axis and (B) short-axis views of the aortic root (arrowheads). C and D, Doppler color flow imaging shows severe aortic insufficiency (arrowheads). E, Using a right transfemoral approach, a 31-mm Medtronic CoreValve (MCV) (Medtronic, Dublin, Ireland) is placed and used to exclude the dissection flap (arrowhead). F, Trivial residual aortic insufficiency is present after placement of the prosthesis. G, Short-axis view of the MCV prosthesis shows exclusion of the aortic dissection flap. Follow-up evaluation performed 2 years after therapy has continued to show normal function of the prosthesis.

Ao, Aortic valve; LA, left atrium; LV, left ventricle; MCV, Medtronic core valve; RA, right atrium; RV, right ventricle.

KEY POINTS

- Transcatheter aortic valve replacement for severe aortic insufficiency remains an area of active investigation.
- In this patient with aortic root dissection and prohibitive surgical risk, transcatheter therapy with a self-expanding prosthesis was acutely effective for treatment of the aortic insufficiency. Anchoring of the self-expanding prosthesis was facilitated by the previously placed interposition graft.

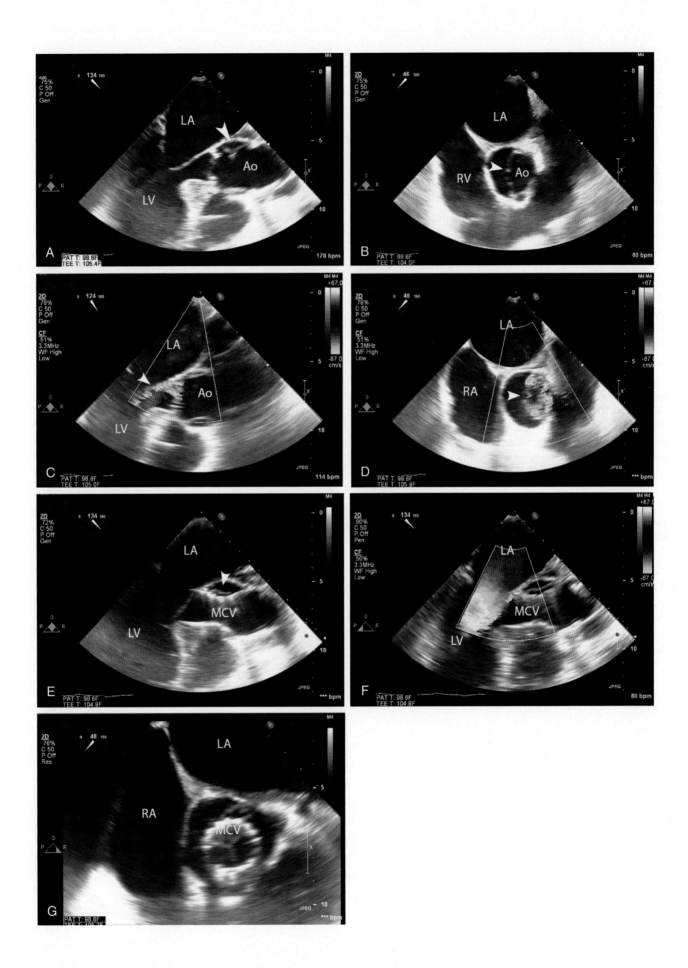

Valve-in-Valve Therapy for Tricuspid Bioprosthetic Failure

Mario Gössl, MD, PhD, Paul Sorajja, MD, and Benjamin Sun, MD

A 50-year-old woman with nonischemic cardiomyopathy, emphysema, and end-stage hypertensive renal disease was found to have severe valvular heart disease, including severe aortic, mitral, and tricuspid valve regurgitation. She underwent surgical replacement of the aortic valve (21-mm Magna Ease bioprosthesis) and the mitral valve (27-mm St. Jude Epic bioprosthesis), as well as tricuspid valve repair with a 32-mm MC3 rigid ring. A, Two months later, she was found to have recurrent severe tricuspid regurgitation as shown on transesophageal echocardiography (TEE) (asterisk). Due to her high surgical risk, she was considered for an off-label, valve-in-tricuspid ring therapy with a transcatheter valve following a thorough heart team discussion. B, The tricuspid ring orifice was sized with computed tomography (CT), and measured 4.9 cm^2 and 30 × 21 mm with an incomplete elliptical shaped tricuspid valve ring. A 29-mm Sapien S3 transcatheter aortic valve (Edwards Lifesciences, Irvine, CA) was chosen for the valve-in-ring therapy. Using right transfemoral vein access, initial attempts using a balloon wedge catheter (Arrow Int., Reading, PA) failed to pass a Lunderquist wire (Cook Medical, Bloomington, IN) due to prolapsing into the right ventricle (RV). Eventually, with support from an 8.5-Fr, Agilis steerable sheath (St. Jude Medical, St. Paul, MN), a stiff Lunderquist wire was placed into the right pulmonary artery. Then, the 29-mm Sapien S3 was deployed within the tricuspid ring using the standard Novaflex delivery system (C, arrow). D, Unfortunately, the percutaneous treatment with the Sapien S3 failed due to severe paravalvular regurgitation (*Sapien S3 frame). E, A 3-Dimensional TEE shows an atrial view of the S3 valve within the tricuspid ring (arrow), and a large medial paravalvular leak (*). The patient ultimately underwent repeat surgery, during which the failure mode of the valve-in-ring therapy was confirmed. F, The transcatheter aortic valve replacement (TAVR) valve-in-ring implantation had pushed the incomplete ring further apart, leading to the severe medial paravalvular regurgitation (dotted line area) next to the TAVR valve (white arrowhead), and the damaged tricuspid ring (white arrow). The Sapien S3 valve and the tricuspid ring were removed, and (G) a 31-mm St. Jude Epic valve was placed with an excellent result (arrow).

KEY POINTS

- The steerable Agilis sheath can help support wire position in difficult cases with wire prolapse into the RV.
- CT is very useful for identification of the appropriate TAVR valve size and implantation angle for valve-in-ring procedures.
- The steerable delivery system of the Edwards Sapien S3 valve can be used to accurately place the TAVR valve within the tricuspid ring, despite acute angulations between right atrium, right ventricle, and pulmonary artery.
- Valve-in-ring procedures can lead to damage of the ring structure, and subsequent paravalvular regurgitation which may require redo-surgery.

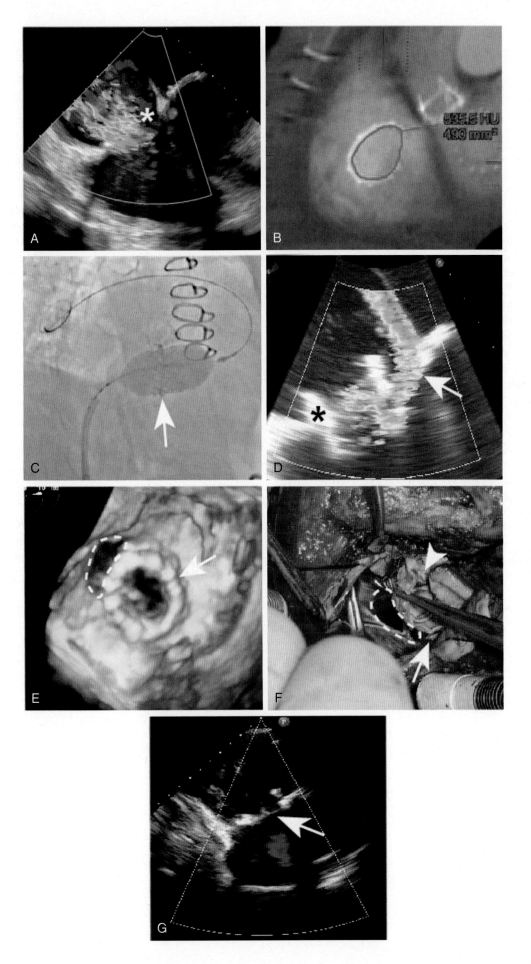

AORTIC VALVE DISEASE 111

Controlled Transcatheter Aortic Valve Replacement

Paul Sorajja, MD

An 84-year-old woman with severe, symptomatic aortic stenosis was referred for catheter-based therapy with the Lotus valve (Boston Scientific, Maple Grove, MN). Preprocedural imaging demonstrated aortic annular dimensions appropriate for a 27-mm prosthesis, with the right iliofemoral system being suitable for access. A, Ascending aortography is performed with a pigtail catheter placed in the noncoronary cusp (arrowhead). With the aortic cups aligned, the target landing zone for the marker on the Lotus valve is the middle of the pigtail catheter. B, A Safari wire (Boston Scientific, Maple Grove, MN) is placed in the left ventricle. This wire, with stiffness for support of the delivery system and a long pre-shaped curve, is specially designed for deployment of the Lotus valve. Balloon aortic valvuloplasty is then performed (not shown). Once the sheathed valve is placed in the thoracic descending aorta, the catheter is rotated to position the marker on the patient's left side (arrowhead) to facilitate passage around the aortic arch. C, The sheathed valve is advanced across the aortic valve, and the operator notes the target landing zone (arrow) for the marker (arrowhead). D, As the valve is unsheathed (arrowhead), the marker (arrow) moves toward the target zone. E, Formation of a waist (arrowhead) helps to determine full apposition of the prosthesis. The valve leaflets are functioning when 50% of the prosthesis is deployed. Note travel of the nosecone along the Safari wire during valve deployment (arrow). F, Ascending aortography is repeated to confirm desired depth for implantation (arrowhead). G, Lay-over of the valve, with placement of the delivery catheter along the greater curvature of the aorta,

is performed to minimize twisting of the posts and thereby facilitate locking of the buckles. The locking is examined with two posts visible as "tuning forks" simultaneously with a third post seen on its side view (arrowheads). The fluoroscopy angle is changed to visualize locking of the third post (not shown). If the operator is not satisfied with positioning or sealing, the prosthesis can be recaptured and repositioned. H, The release pin (arrowhead) is removed. At this point, the valve can still be retrieved. I, Aortography shows no paravalvular regurgitation following compete deployment. J, Final image of the Lotus prosthesis on fluoroscopy (arrowhead).

Ao, Ascending aorta; LV, left ventricle; Pig, pigtail catheter.

KEY POINTS

- The Lotus valve is placed with slow, controlled expansion of the prosthesis at the target zone, and without the need for rapid ventricular pacing.
- A complete assessment of the final valve position, hemodynamics, and presence of any paravalvular regurgitation can be performed with the ability to fully recapture and reposition the prosthesis if desired.

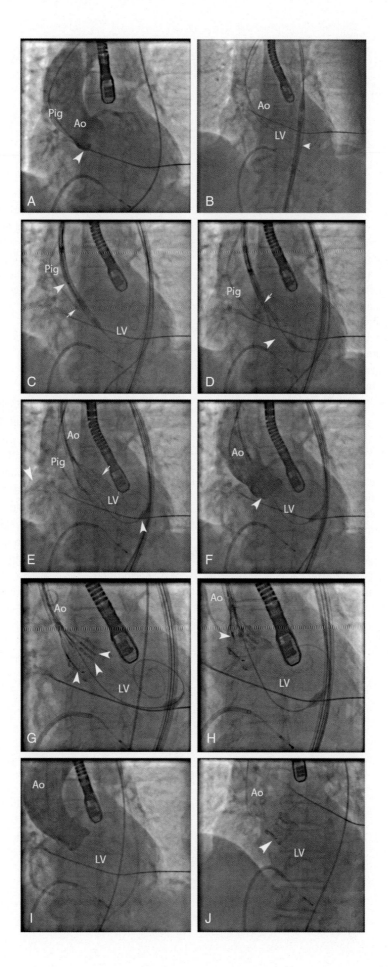

Left Ventricular Perforation During Transcatheter Aortic Valve Replacement

Paul Sorajja, MD

An 87-year-old man was hospitalized with decompensated heart failure due to severe aortic stenosis. Preprocedural imaging demonstrated severe stenosis with a tricuspid valve, and suitable iliofemoral arteries for a transcatheter approach. A, Following routine crossing of the aortic valve (arrow), a pigtail catheter was placed and then used to exchange for a 0.038″ Amplatz Super Stiff guidewire (Boston Scientific, Marlborough, MA). This diastolic frame shows the initial positioning of the wire, which had been manuall shaped (arrowhead). A temporary pacemaker (TPM) was placed from the right femoral vein through an 8-Fr Mullins sheath, which helps to provide stability during rapid ventricular pacing. B, During systole, kinking of the stiff guidewire is seen with an acute angle of the wire directed toward the left ventricular free wall (arrowhead). C, During balloon valvuloplasty, one can see further distortion of the guidewire with creation of a more abrupt transition (arrowhead). D, Malposition of the wire remains during deployment of a 26-mm Sapien XT (Edwards Lifesciences, Irving, CA). One hour after completion of the procedure, the patient begins to have hypotension that is refractory to intravenous fluids and vasoactive medications. Emergent echocardiography demonstrates a pericardial effusion (asterisk) on apical long-axis (E) and parasternal short-axis (F) imaging with tamponade physiology and coagulum (arrowheads). The pericardial effusion is refractory to pericardiocentesis. The patient undergoes emergency surgery, where a wire exit perforation in the lateral ventricular wall is identified. Despite successful repair, the patient dies of multi-organ failure several days later.

Ao, Ascending aorta; AV, aortic valve; BAV, balloon valvuloplasty; LV, left ventricle; RV, right ventricle; SG, Swan-Ganz catheter; TEE, transesophageal echocardiography; TPM, temporary pacemaker.

KEY POINTS

- Use of a supportive guidewire with a long, gradual transition toward the stiff segment is an essential part of transcatheter aortic valve replacement. When manually-shaping the guidewire, it is essential to avoid abrupt transitions.
- Pre-shaped, exchange-length guidewires (Safari, Boston Scientific, Maple Grove, MN; Confida, Medtronic, Coon Rapids, MN), while more costly than traditional wires, are commonly used and can help reduce the risk of wire exit and left ventricular perforation.

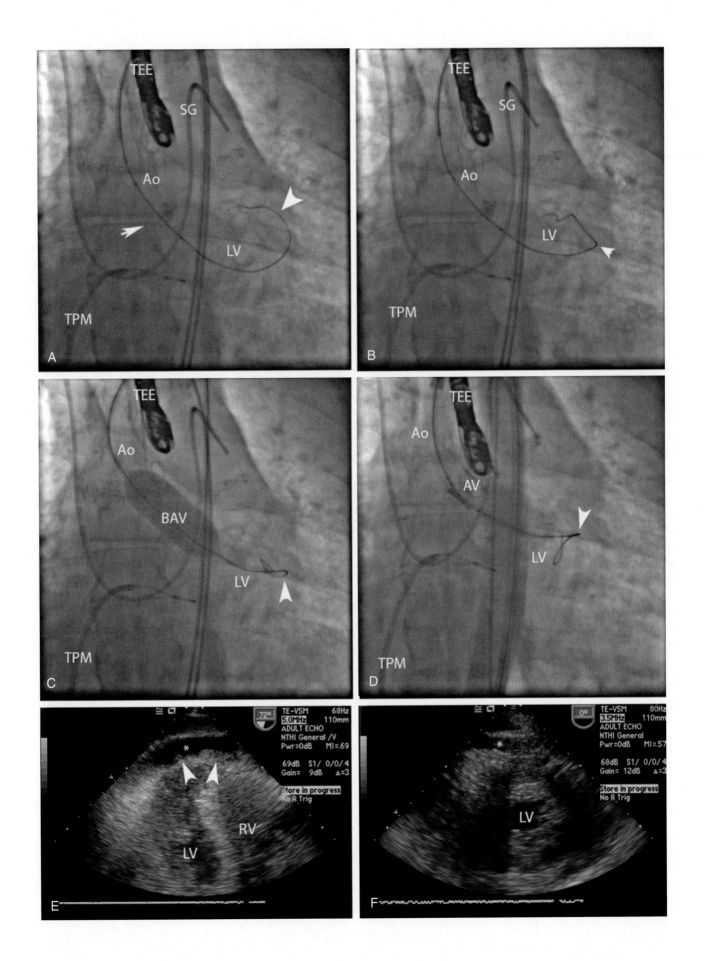

Transcatheter Aortic Valve Replacement for Subaortic Ring Treatment

Norihiko Kamioka, MD, Ateet Patel, MD, Stamatios Lerakis, MD, Ioannis Parastatidis, MD, Jessica Forcillo, MD, Frank Corrigan, MD, Vinod H. Thourani, MD, Peter Block, MD, and Vasilis Babaliaros, MD

A 34-year-old woman with Down's syndrome had a history of an atrioventricular canal repair. In addition, 11 years ago she underwent a subaortic membrane resection and a mechanical mitral valve (MV) replacement. She came to our hospital with worsening symptoms of heart failure. A, Transthoracic echocardiography identified recurrent discrete subaortic stenosis (SAS) (arrowhead) with the mean gradient of 67 mm Hg. B, Multidetector computed tomography (MDCT) confirmed subaortic stenosis (arrow) beneath the aortic annular plane (broken line). Because of her significant cognitive impairment and two prior sternotomies, she was deemed a poor surgical candidate. Transcatheter treatment, using the same technique as transcatheter aortic valve replacement (TAVR), was planned for SAS. MDCT revealed her arterial access was inadequate for traditional transfemoral access or subclavian access. Therefore, the procedure was performed via transcaval access.

The procedure was done under general anesthesia in the catheterization laboratory. C, MDCT imaging suggested the aorta adjacent to the top of the second lumbar vertebra was suitable for the puncture point (arrowhead). D, An energized Confianza Pro guidewire (Abbott Vascular, Santa Clara, CA) (arrow) was crossed from the inferior vena cava (IVC) into the aorta toward a snare catheter (arrowhead) and was subsequently exchanged for a Lunderquist wire (Cook, Bloomington, IN). After the establishment of transcaval access, a 14-Fr sheath was advanced from the right femoral vein into the aorta. E, A 20-mm balloon valvuloplasty was done first, and identified the plane of the subaortic stenosis from its indentation during balloon inflation (yellow line), relative to the plane of the aortic annulus identified by the pigtail catheter (white dashed line). F, A 23-mm Sapien 3 valve (Edwards Lifesciences, Irvine, CA) was then deployed spanning the plane of the subaortic stenosis (yellow line) and the aortic annulus (white dashed line). This deployment relieved the subaortic stenosis (arrowhead) without paravalvular leakage and without interfering with the mechanical MV function. G, The mean transaortic gradient had fallen to 12 mm Hg. H, The aorto-caval fistula was closed with a 10/8-mm Amplatzer Duct Occluder (arrow; St. Jude Medical, St. Paul, MN). The patient was discharged with symptom relief on postoperative day 1. At follow-up 1 year later, the gradient remains unchanged and the patient has resolution of heart failure.

KEY POINTS

- Transcatheter treatment for subaortic stenosis can be performed in patients with high surgical risk.
- In patients with inadequate vascular access for arterial transfemoral TAVR, transcaval to aortic access can be used as an alternative strategy.
- Balloon valvuloplasty before valve implantation is an adjunctive method for sizing of the subaortic stenosis, as well as confirmation of the location of the stenosis.

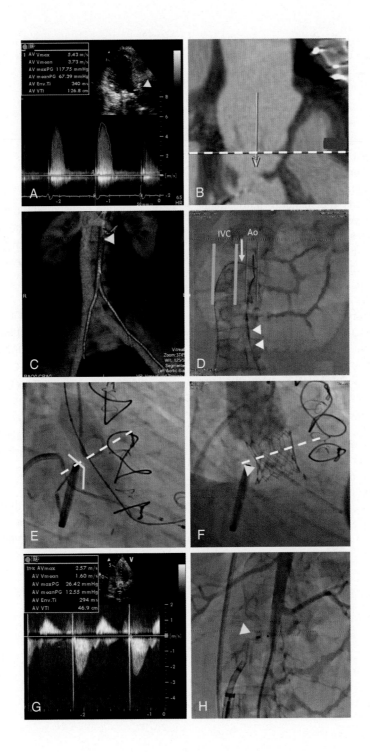

Bicuspid Aortic Valve Therapy Transcatheter Challenges

Nay M. Htun, MBBS, MRCP (UK), FRACP, PhD, and John Graydon Webb, MD

A 70-year-old man with past a history of liver cirrhosis, ischemic cardiomyopathy, and dual chamber pacemaker, presented with exertional dyspnea secondary to severe aortic stenosis. He was referred for transfemoral transcatheter aortic valve replacement (TAVR). A and B, Transthoracic echocardiography demonstrates a severely calcified, bicuspid aortic valve (A, parasternal short-axis view; B, parasternal long-axis view) with a (C) mean gradient of 45 mm Hg. D, Computed tomography of the aortic valve shows type 1A bicuspid morphology (the commonest variant) with the fusion of left and right coronary cusps (arrow). Aortography of bicuspid aortic stenosis (E) lacks the classic orthogonal view usually seen in tricuspid aortic valves (F). The aortic valve is crossed using a left Amplatz catheter and a straight wire, which is then exchanged for a 0.035″ extra-stiff wire with a large pigtail-shaped curve. G, The SAPIEN 3 (S3) (Edwards Lifesciences, Irvine, CA) is positioned with the middle marker underlying the bioprosthesis just above the plane of the angiographic annulus. H, The transcatheter heart valve (THV) is deployed under rapid ventricular pacing. The mean gradient across the bioprosthesis is 6 mm Hg and there is only trivial aortic regurgitation post-TAVR.

KEY POINTS

- Although bicuspid aortic valves are common, TAVR has been relatively contraindicated in these patients due to complex anatomy, including eccentric and heavy calcification of leaflets, calcified raphe, and associated aortopathy with horizontal and dilated aorta.
- Angiographic appearance of aortic cusps in bicuspid valves can be irregular and asymmetric due to the lack of classic orthogonal view seen in tricuspid aortic valves. Hence, crossing the stenotic bicuspid valve and achieving ideal implantation heights of THVs can be challenging.
- Newer generation THVs with external sealing skirts have been shown to have less paravalvular regurgitation in bicuspid aortic cases, compared to the relatively high incidence associated with older generation devices.
- Permanent pacemaker implantation rate after TAVR is higher in patients with bicuspid aortic valves, highlighting the importance of optimal positioning of THVs.

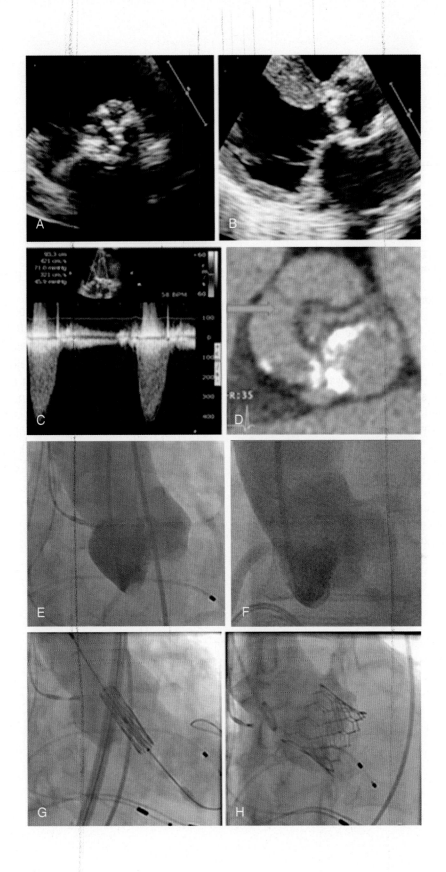

Transcatheter Aortic Valve-in-Valve Therapy With High Risk of Coronary Obstruction

Itsik Ben-Dor, MD, Zuyue Wang, MD, Ron Waksman, MD, Lowell Satler, MD, and Augusto Pichard, MD

An 89-year-old woman with dyspnea is referred for transcatheter aortic valve replacement. She previously underwent coronary artery bypass grafting and aortic valve replacement with a Mitroflow Synergy 21-mm prosthesis (Sorin Group, Milan, Italy). A–C, Echocardiography demonstrated bioprosthetic valve failure with severe stenosis, with an aortic valve area of 0.5 cm^2, peak aortic velocity of 3.8 m/s, and a mean gradient of 33 mm Hg. Computed tomography (CT) showed long Mitroflow leaflets extend beyond the coronary ostia. Coronary protection was performed with two 5-Fr guiding catheters, both placed from the right femoral artery. For the left coronary artery, an EBU 3.5 guide was used to position a 3.5 × 18 mm Xience stent (Abbott Vascular, Santa Clara, CA) in the left anterior descending artery. D, In the right coronary artery, a hockey stick guide was used to place a 3.0 × 15 mm Xience stent. E, A 23-mm Sapien XT (Edwards Lifesciences, Irving, CA) was delivered transfemorally from the left groin and deployed during rapid pacing. F, After valve deployment coronary flow was normal in left and right coronaries: both stents were pulled back into the aorta. G, Final aortography showed no aortic regurgitation and normal coronary flow. The mean gradient across the aortic valve was 12 mm Hg.

KEY POINTS

- Coronary obstruction following transcatheter aortic valve replacement is a rare (0.66%), but life-threatening complication.
- On CT, a low origin of the coronary ostia (<12 mm) and a narrow aortic root (<30 mm) are important risk factors for coronary obstruction.
- Stentless valves, with externally mounted leaflets, and valves with supra-annular positioning pose the highest risk for coronary obstruction.
- For patients with significantly increased risk of coronary obstruction, protection of the arteries can be performed with preemptive placement of coronary guidewires and stent distal to the ostia.

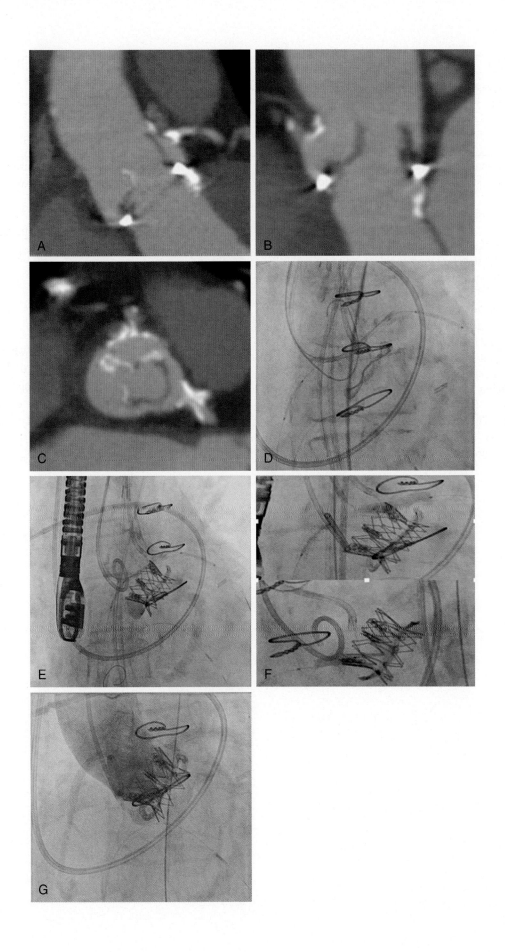

A Difficult Case of Transcatheter Aortic Valve Replacement

Brandon M. Jones, MD, Stephanie Mick, MD, and Samir R. Kapadia, MD

An 83-year-old man presented with progressive dyspnea and severe aortic stenosis in the setting of prior thoracic endovascular aortic repair for type B aortic dissection. The patient was considered to be high surgical risk due to age and comorbidities, and transcatheter aortic valve replacement was undertaken. Several procedural challenges were present: (A and B) the stent graft would need to be carefully traversed; (C) the patient had a horizontal ascending aorta; (D) there was partial fusion of the right and noncoronary cusps, posing challenges for valve sizing and the potential for paravalvular regurgitation; and (E) there was an annular area of 438 mm^2, which is borderline for choosing a 23-mm or a 26-mm Edwards S3 prosthesis (Edwards Lifesciences, Irvine, CA). F, To address these challenges, we first started with balloon sizing of the aortic annulus using a 23 mm × 4 cm ES balloon (Edwards Lifesciences) and simultaneous aortography. There was severe regurgitation during full balloon expansion, but adequate space in the sinus of Valsalva. Thus we chose a 26-mm Edwards S3 device. G, A major benefit of the S3 is the ability to use active flexion of the distal portion of the Commander delivery system, which assists with traversing the endograft, as well as hyperflexion during positioning in the horizontal aorta during valve implantation. H, Final aortography demonstrated satisfactory positioning of the S3 prosthesis.

KEY POINTS

- Balloon sizing can be an effective way to select the appropriate valve prosthesis in borderline cases.
- In horizontal aorta cases, the ability to flex the distal portion of the Commander delivery sheath can assist with coaxial alignment of the valve to the aortic annular plane.

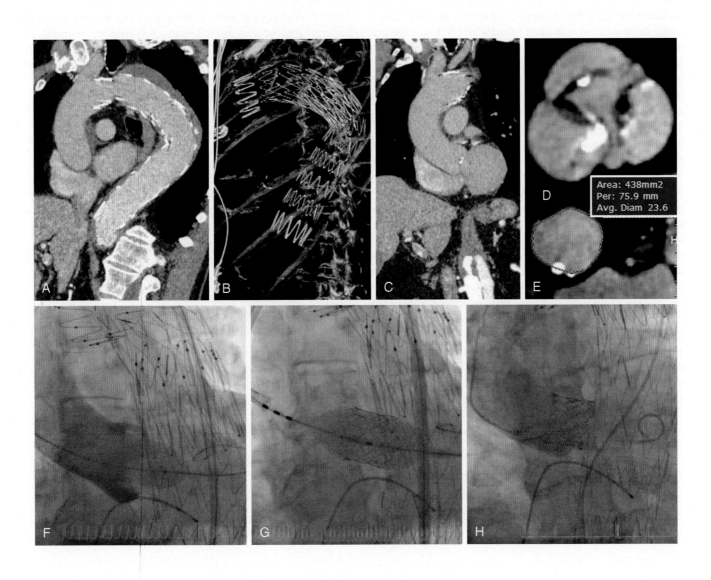

Valve Embolization During Transcatheter Aortic Valve Therapy

Judit Karacsonyi, MD, Shuaib Abdullah, MD, Imre Ungi, MD, PhD, Ravi Joshi, MD, Subhash Banerjee, MD, and Emmanouil S. Brilakis, MD, PhD

An 82-year-old man with high-risk, severe aortic valve stenosis was referred for elective transcatheter aortic valve replacement (TAVR). Echocardiography revealed severe aortic valve stenosis with peak velocity of 4.0 m/s, mean gradient of 40 mm Hg, and aortic valve area of 1 cm² with mild regurgitation. The aortic valve area was calcified and possibly bicuspid (A), with an area of 507 mm². A 6-Fr pigtail catheter was advanced into the aortic valve cusps via the left femoral artery. Over a manually pre-shaped Lunderquist guidewire, a 23-mm Edwards balloon (Edwards Lifesciences, Irvine, CA) was inflated across the aortic valve to eliminate the waist. Simultaneous aortography demonstrated adequate sealing without significant regurgitation. A 26-mm Edwards Sapien XT valve prosthesis (Edwards Lifesciences) was carefully positioned and deployed during held ventilation and rapid pacing (B, arrow). Following placement, there was moderate aortic regurgitation and post-dilation was performed with the implant balloon. Final angiography (C, arrow) and transesophageal echocardiography (TEE) revealed optimal valve positioning with mild regurgitation (E and F, arrow). Following closure of the arterial access sites, widening of the QRS duration occurred without hemodynamic instability. Repeat TEE revealed downward displacement of the valve (G, arrow), which was not clearly identifiable on fluoroscopy (D, arrow). A decision was made to attempt to cross the valve prosthesis with a wire. After multiple attempts, the guidewire was advanced across the native aortic valve. The tip of the guidewire then touched the frame of the prosthesis, followed by displacement of the prosthesis into the left ventricle (H, arrow). The patient was placed emergently on bypass using arterial and venous cannulations, followed by removal of the TAVR prosthesis and implantation of a 25-mm Edwards Perimount Magna Ease valve (Edwards Lifesciences). The patient recovered well from the operation.

Ao, Ascending aorta; LA, left atrium; LV, left ventricle.

KEY POINTS

- Embolization of prostheses during TAVR is a rare and life-threatening complication. Potential causes of embolization include positioning error, lack of calcification, and use of undersized prostheses.
- Embolization into the aorta is easier to manage than loss of the prosthesis into the left ventricle. In all instances, obtaining and/or maintaining wire access across the prosthesis is essential to maintain normal antegrade flow.
- For left ventricular embolization, emergent conversion to open cardiac surgery is the main method of correction.

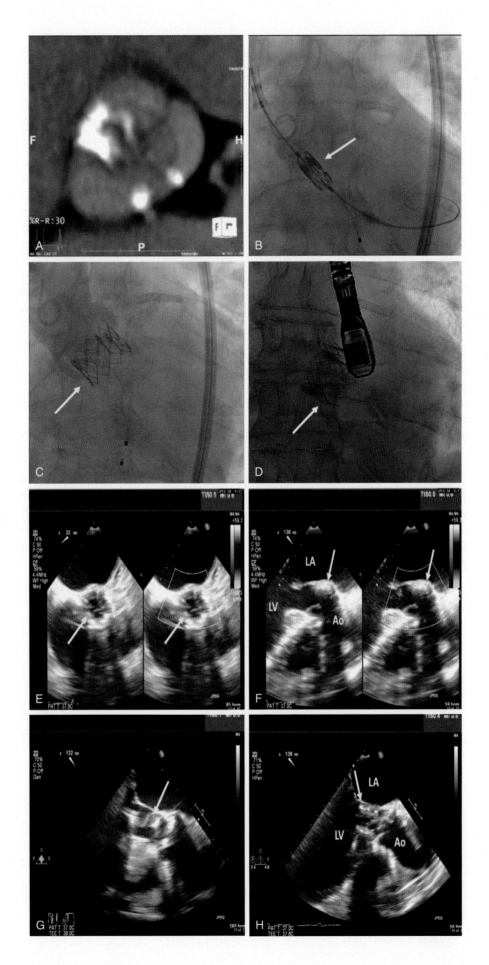

Transcaval Transcatheter Aortic Valve Replacement

John J. Kelly, BA, Vasilis Babaliaros, MD, and Vinod H. Thourani, MD

A frail 88-year-old woman with severe aortic stenosis and multiple comorbidities was referred for transcatheter aortic valve replacement (TAVR). Computed tomography (CT) revealed femoral arteries too small for the transfemoral arterial approach, and thus transcaval access was selected. CT with 3-dimensional modeling was used to identify a calcification-free window of the abdominal aorta, located >15 mm below the renal arteries and >15 mm above the aortic bifurcation, for the creation of a transcaval fistula between the aorta and inferior vena cava (IVC). A level just superior to the L3 vertebral body was selected (A–D).

Under general anesthesia, both femoral veins and the right femoral artery were accessed. A single-loop snare was positioned in the abdominal aorta through a 6-Fr guiding catheter. A railing catheter system consisting of a coronary guidewire (0.014″ × 300 cm), a locking wire converter (0.035″ × 145 cm), and a microcatheter (0.035″ × 90 cm) telescoped inside a 6-Fr renal length internal mammary guiding catheter was positioned in the IVC. The external end of the guidewire was attached to electrocautery using a hemostat. Once correct device positioning was confirmed with biplane fluoroscopy, the guidewire was electrified at 50W, cut, and advanced from the IVC to the snare in the aorta (E–G). This fistula was progressively dilated as the wire converter and microcatheter were advanced. These were exchanged for an extra-stiff guidewire (0.035″ × 260 cm), over which the 14-Fr valve sheath was introduced. TAVR was then performed with a 23-mm Sapien 3 valve (Edwards Lifesciences, Irvine, CA) without complication (H).

Following TAVR, the transcaval fistula was closed with an Amplatzer 10/8 duct occluder (Abbot Vascular, Santa Clara, CA; I). There was no extravasation of contrast on final angiography (J). The patient was extubated immediately after the procedure, and was discharged on postoperative day 2. At 30-day follow-up, she had no complaints and was in New York Heart Association class I. Echocardiography showed excellent transcatheter valve function with mean gradient of 8 mm Hg, and there was no residual aorto-caval fistula on follow-up abdominal CT.

IVC, Inferior vena cava.

KEY POINTS

- The transcaval approach is a viable alternative for patients who are unable to undergo transfemoral arterial TAVR. In this procedure, preoperative planning with the Heart Team to develop an optimal treatment strategy for each patient is essential.

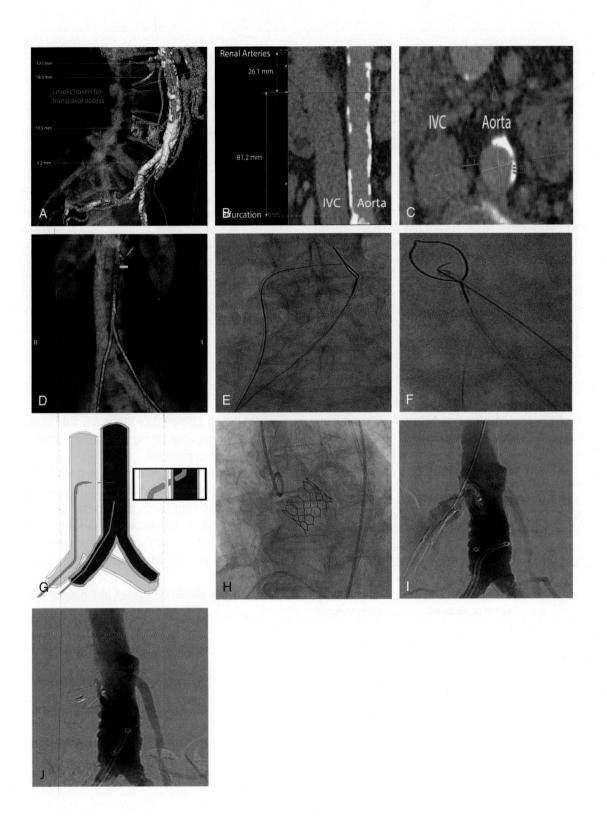

Subclavian Management During Transcatheter Aortic Valve Replacement

Hasan Ahmad, MD, and Gilbert H. L. Tang, MD, MSc, MBA

A 50-year-old woman with severe aortic stenosis and end-stage renal disease on hemodialysis was referred for transcatheter aortic valve replacement (TAVR). A, A 26-mm Edwards Sapien 3 prosthesis (Edwards Lifesciences, Irvine, CA) was chosen on the basis of an annulus area of 469.7 mm^2 with a mean annulus diameter of 24.6 mm. The iliofemoral arteries were inadequate for vascular access, and alternate access sites were evaluated. B, Three-dimensional reconstruction and cross-sectional imaging with computed tomography indicated that the left subclavian artery (LSA) was appropriate, based on size and angulation of the ascending aorta and native aortic valve. C, The distance from the left axillary arteriotomy (LAA) site to the aortic annulus and to the mid ascending aorta was measured, and marked on the 14-FR Edwards eSheath. D, The LSA was prewired with a 0.018″ V-18 ControlWire (Boston Scientific, Maple Grove, MN), which had been placed from a 7-Fr sheath in the left femoral artery. E, Following cut-down to the LAA, the aortic valve was crossed in standard fashion, followed by placement of a Lunderquist wire (Cook Medical, Bloomington, IN) in the left ventricle. The Edwards eSheath dilator was pre-curved, flushed, and lubricated with propofol. The eSheath, with the sleeve opening facing the patient's face and the Edwards logo facing the patient's feet, was then gradually advanced to the mid-ascending aorta. F, To minimize movement of the eSheath and injury to the LSA, a balloon aortic valvuloplasty was performed, followed by passage of a propofol-lubricated Commander system to just above the annulus. G, The Sapien 3 valve was loaded onto the balloon in the ascending aorta, advanced across the aortic annulus, and deployed with rapid ventricular pacing. H, After confirming proper deployment, the delivery system was withdrawn and the dilator was reintroduced into the eSheath, followed by gradual removal as a unit over the stiff wire. I, Following surgical repair of the arteriotomy, a completion angiogram of the LSA was performed to ensure the integrity before withdrawing the V-18 wire.

KEY POINTS

- For cases where injury to the left subclavian artery may occur, pre-wiring from the femoral artery should be considered.
- To help minimize risk of injury to the left subclavian artery, consider noting the sheath markers to facilitate monitoring of its movement, utilize propofol for lubrication, introduce the eSheath with the slit facing the head and the Edwards logo facing the feet, and remove the system over the stiff wire as a unit.
- The valve should be loaded in the ascending aorta.

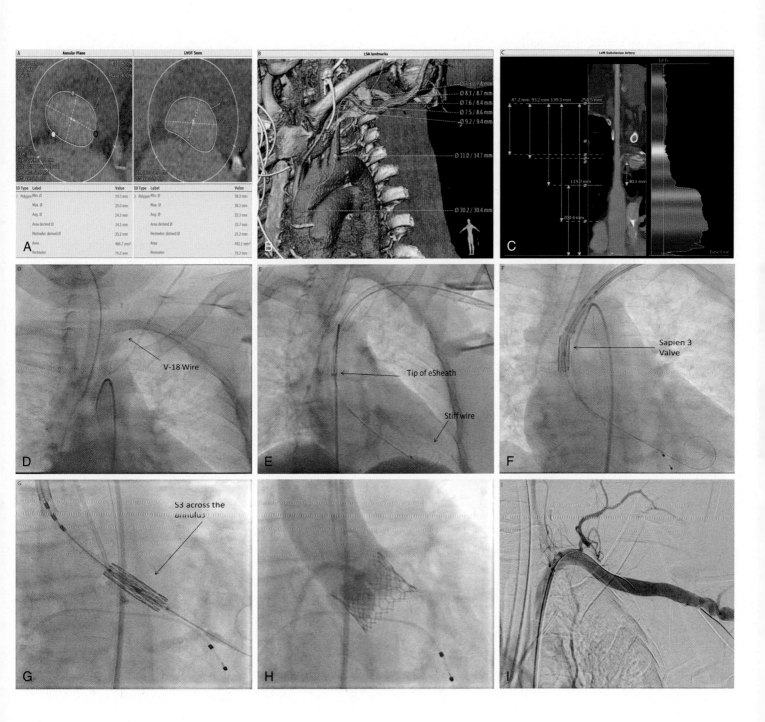

Rapid Ventricular Pacing and Demise of Ventricular Function

Paul Sorajja, MD

A 77-year-old woman is brought to the cardiac catheterization laboratory for transcatheter aortic valve replacement (TAVR) for the treatment of severe, calcific aortic stenosis. The patient had no history of coronary artery disease; her left ventricular function was normal with an ejection fraction of 62%. A, Baseline transesophageal echocardiogram (TEE) with 3-dimensional (3-D) imaging shows a competent mitral valve (MV) with full apposition of the valve leaflets at end-systole. B, Short-axis imaging of the AV demonstrates calcific stenosis. C, A 260-cm, pre-shaped Safari wire (arrow; Boston Scientific, Maple Grove, MN) (arrowhead) is placed into the left ventricle. Rapid ventricular pacing at 180 bpm for 6 seconds is performed during balloon aortic valvuloplasty using a 18/23-mm V8 balloon (Intervalve, Minnetonka, MN). The patient's blood pressure does not recover after pacing is stopped, and remains 40/0 mm Hg. D, TEE with 3-D imaging shows acute left ventricular dilatation and an incompetent MV (arrow). E, Acute severe mitral regurgitation (arrowhead) is present. F, A 26-mm Sapien S3 (Edwards Lifesciences, Irving, CA) is quickly placed (arrowhead), followed by chest compressions for 30 seconds and intravenous administration of epinephrine. G and H, Within 5 min, the patient's left ventricular function returns to normal and the MV becomes competent again, with only mild residual MR (arrowhead). The patient recovered fully, without neurological deficits, and was discharged after an otherwise uneventful hospital stay.

Ao, Aorta; AV, aortic valve; LA, left atrium; MV, mitral valve; RA, right atrium; RV, right ventricle.

KEY POINTS

- Rapid ventricular pacing may cause acute left ventricular dysfunction and hemodynamic compromise. Patients with and without underlying ischemic heart disease may be vulnerable to this phenomenon.
- When severe hypotension is present during TAVR, rapid treatment of the aortic stenosis with placement of the prosthesis can be life-saving.

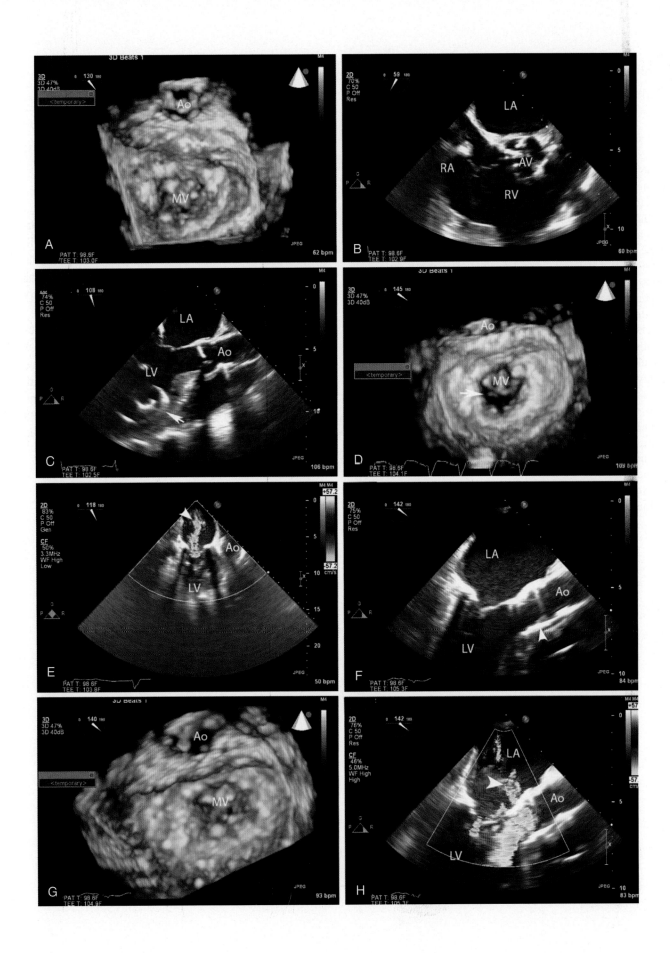

Pure Aortic Regurgitation Treatment

Cameron Dowling, MBBS, and Stephen Brecker, MD

A 66-year-old woman with symptomatic, severe aortic valve regurgitation was referred for transcatheter aortic valve replacement (TAVR). She had a history of radiotherapy for Hodgkin's lymphoma, complicated by radiation-induced coronary artery disease. Twelve years ago, she had undergone coronary artery bypass grafting with subsequent mediastinitis and delayed wound healing. For these reasons, a transcatheter approach was chosen. A–C, Procedural transesophageal echocardiography (TEE) and aortography revealed a trileaflet aortic valve with minimal calcification. The leaflets were retracted, resulting in severe central aortic regurgitation (arrow) with a wide pulse pressure. D, The aortic annulus diameter was 21.6 mm. A 26-mm Medtronic CoreValve (arrow; Mounds View, MN) was chosen to achieve 20% oversizing. No balloon predilatation was performed. The valve was deployed under rapid pacing to minimize hemodynamic instability and stabilize valve positioning. E–H, Post-deployment aortography, TEE, and hemodynamic tracings demonstrated only trivial paravalvular leak (arrows; F and G).

Ao, Ascending aorta; CV, CoreValve prosthesis; LA, left atrium; LV, left ventricle.

KEY POINTS

- The lack of aortic leaflet calcification poses significant challenges for valve positioning in TAVR. Repeated aortograms can help define the aortic root anatomy. In some cases, the use of two pigtail catheters, positioned in the non- and right-coronary cusps, may be utilized.
- For anchoring, up to 25% oversizing may be required. Deployment under rapid pacing decreases the regurgitant fraction and helps stabilize the valve position. Balloon predilatation is not recommended.
- For added potential effectiveness and safety, one may consider use of a recapturable valve with a sealing skirt (for example, Medtronic CoreValve Evolut PRO).

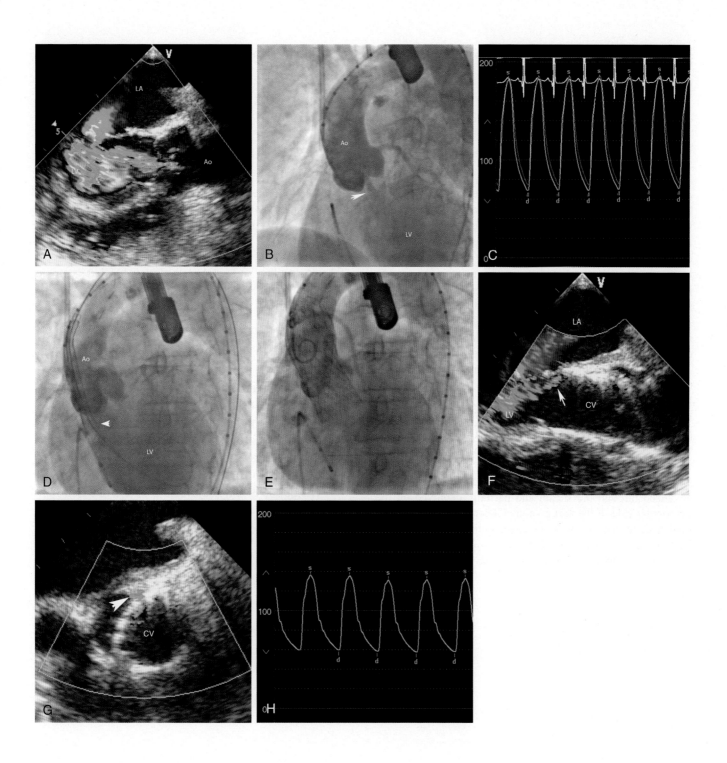

Percutaneous Closure of Aortic Valve for Persistent Aortic Insufficiency With Left Ventricular Assist Device

Joseph M. Venturini, MD, and Atman P. Shah, MD

A 69-year-old man with history of ischemic cardiomyopathy requiring left ventricular assist device (LVAD) support was referred for percutaneous transcatheter closure of the aortic valve. Transesophageal echocardiography (TEE) demonstrated central aortic insufficiency (arrowheads) in (A) long-axis and (B) short-axis view. The dimensions for the left ventricular outflow tract and sinuses of Valsalva measured to be 24 mm and 30 mm, respectively, on TEE. C, Aortography confirmed the significant aortic insufficiency in the setting of the LVAD inflow cannula noted on fluoroscopy (asterisk). D, The aortic valve was crossed with a 6-Fr AL1 catheter stiff, followed by placement of an Amplatzer 0.035″ × 260 cm guidewire (St. Jude Medical, St. Paul, MN), which was advanced and looped in the apex of the left ventricle. An 8-Fr Amplatzer TorqVue delivery sheath (St. Jude Medical, St. Paul, MN) (arrow) was advanced retrograde over the guidewire into the left ventricle (asterisks) under echocardiographic guidance. E, A 30-mm Amplatzer Cribriform Occluder (St. Jude Medical, St. Paul, MN) was advanced through the sheath and partially deployed on the ventricular side of the aortic valve. Under echocardiographic guidance, the device was retracted against the ventricular side of the aortic valve (arrowhead). F and G, The proximal disc was then exposed on the aortic side of the aortic valve (arrowheads) under echocardiographic (F) and fluoroscopic (G) guidance. After confirming adequate seating of the device and no significant valvular regurgitation, the device was deployed. H, Postprocedural TEE in long-axis demonstrated no residual regurgitation.

Ao, Ascending aorta; LA, left atrium; LV, left ventricle; RA, right atrium; RV, right ventricle.

KEY POINTS

- Following retrograde placement of the Cribiform device, the occluder is fully deployed across the valve but not released immediately. Prolonged hemodynamic monitoring (>10 min) with the device in place may be necessary to fully assess the hemodynamic effects of aortic valve closure. The device is fully retrievable until it is released.
- Measurement of the aortic valve annulus area with TEE can be used to facilitate appropriate sizing of the occluder device.

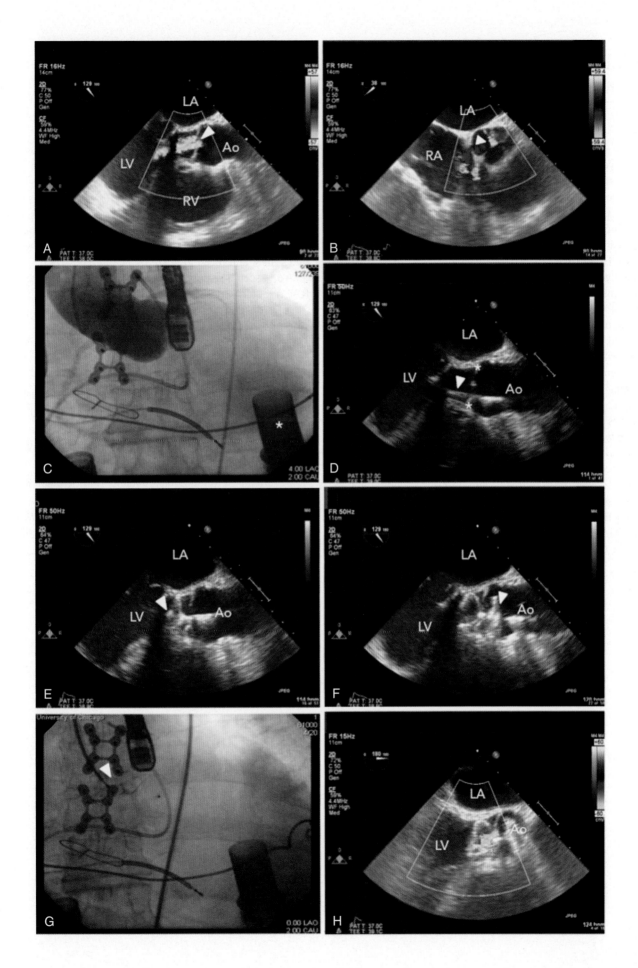

Recurrent Valve Thrombus Early and Late After TAVR

John R. Lesser, MD

A 79-year-old man presented with symptomatic, severe aortic stenosis and underwent uncomplicated, transfemoral placement of a 23-mm Sapien S3 (Edwards Lifesciences, Irvine, CA). He was in sinus rhythm and treated with dual antiplatelet therapy. The postprocedural echocardiogram showed a peak aortic velocity of 2.7 m/s and a mean gradient of 13 mm Hg. Two days after valve placement, cardiac computed tomography (CT) demonstrated hypoattenuated low-density tissue (HALT; presumed thrombus) (A) at the base of the leaflets (arrows, short-axis in diastole), but (B) not involving the leaflet tips (short-axis in diastole). C and D, Mild leaflet restriction was noted with cine CT (C, arrow in short-axis view; D, arrow in long-axis view). E and F, Warfarin was initiated, and the HALT resolved on the next imaging scans at 1 and 4 months (E, short-axis at leaflet base; F, long-axis in diastole). There were no corresponding changes in aortic hemodynamics on echocardiography. Coumadin was discontinued after 6 months followed by initiation of aspirin. A repeat echocardiogram performed at 9 months postprocedure showed a peak aortic velocity of 3.4 m/s and a mean gradient of 26 mm Hg, with no clear structural abnormality seen on two-dimensional echocardiographic imaging. G and H, Repeat cardiac CT demonstrated recurrent, prominent HALT involving 2 of the 3 leaflets (G, arrows, short axis in diastole; H, arrows, long axis in diastole). I and J,

Additionally, there was prominent restriction in leaflet motion (I, arrows, short-axis systolic imaging; J, arrows, long-axis systolic imaging) on cine CT. Warfarin was reinitiated and continued indefinitely. At 1-year post-transcatheter aortic valve replacement, the aortic hemodynamics on echocardiography returned to baseline with a peak aortic velocity of 2.2 m/s, and mean gradient of 11 mm Hg.

Ao, Ascending aorta; LA, left atrium; LV, left ventricle; RA, right atrium; RV, right ventricle.

KEY POINTS

- The timing and occurrence of HALT has varying onset and is best visualized with a cardiac CT angiography.
- The imaging of the valve leaflets and aortic valve gradients on transthoracic echocardiography may remain unremarkable despite the presence of HALT.
- The presumed thrombus often resolves with warfarin initiation but may recur with drug discontinuation.

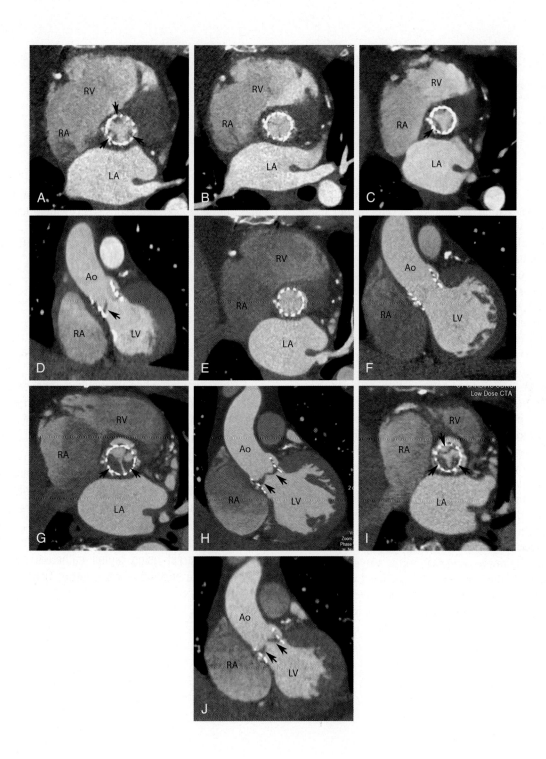

Transcatheter Aortic Valve Therapy Without Preprocedural Computed Tomography

Paul Sorajja, MD

A 62-year-old man was hospitalized for congestive heart failure, in the setting of known severe aortic stenosis. Although he was initially medically stable, the patient became unstable and dependent on inotropic support. A, Initially, bridging balloon valvuloplasty was considered, but there was moderately-severe aortic regurgitation (arrow). B, Using 3-dimensional imaging on transesophageal echocardiography, the aortic valve area was measured to be 4.26 cm^2 with a perimeter of 73 mm. C, Peripheral intravascular ultrasound (arrow) was performed over a super stiff wire to examine tortuosity and peripheral artery dimensions. D, On intravascular ultrasound, the minimal lumen diameter was 10.2 mm. E, A 26-mm Evolut R prosthesis (Ev; Medtronic, St. Paul, MN) (arrowhead) was chosen and positioned with the help of a pigtail catheter placed from the left femoral artery. F, The prosthetic valve was initially underexpanded due to the severe aortic valve calcification (arrowhead). G, Immediately after deployment, there was severe paravalvular regurgitation on echocardiography (arrowhead). I, Following post-dilatation with a 21/26 mm V8 balloon (InterValve, Minnetonka, MN), (H) there was only trivial degree of paravalvular regurgitation (arrow), and (J) the inflow of the valve was fully expanded (arrowhead). K, Preprocedural invasive hemodynamics showed a mean aortic valve gradient of 84 mm Hg. L, Following placement of the Evolut R prosthesis and post-dilatation, the mean aortic valve gradient was 5 mm Hg. Note the significant decrease in the left ventricular end-diastolic pressure and widening of the aortic-ventricular diastolic pressure gap, consistent with alleviation of the aortic regurgitation.

Ao, Ascending aorta; Ev, Evolut R; LV, left ventricle; Pig, pigtail catheter.

KEY POINTS

- Transcatheter aortic valve replacement can be performed without preprocedural computed tomography when meticulous echocardiographic assessment of the valve area and peripheral intravascular ultrasound is employed. The aortic valve area should be measured with 3-dimensional imaging.
- In situations with uncertain aortic dimensions, the use of the Evolut R prosthesis is advantageous due to its ability to be recaptured in the event that a sizing error occurs.
- The procedure can be performed completely with no contrast using pigtail catheters positioned in both the noncoronary and left coronary aortic valve cusps.

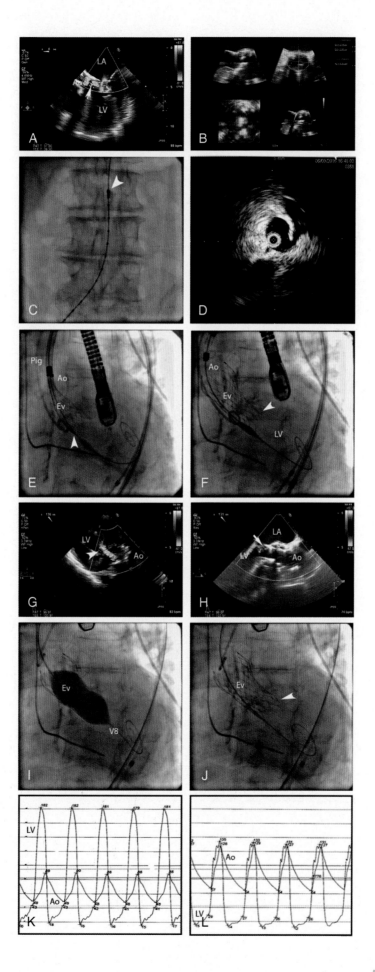

Prosthetic Valve

Cardiac Computed Tomography Evaluation of a Paravalvular Leak

John R. Lesser, MD

A 76-year-old man, who previously underwent surgery with a 23-mm Trifecta prosthesis (St. Jude Medical, St. Paul, MN), presented with severe paravalvular aortic insufficiency (AI). Cardiac computed tomography (CT) was performed in order to help with procedural planning for percutaneous closure. The acquisition encompassed a full function dataset with thin slices for the intervals that best stopped cardiac motion. Echocardiographic images were reviewed to identify the orientation that best showed the exit of the AI jet. A, The region on the CT that corresponded to the Doppler signal of AI was interrogated for paravalvular regurgitation, which was seen well on a transthoracic apical 5-chamber view. B, On CT, the same view was obtained to identify the paravalvular regurgitation (arrow). C, Similarly, the paravalvular regurgitation site is first identified on transesophageal echocardiography (arrow), and (D) this corresponded to the imaging plane on CT to identify the site of paravalvular regurgitation (arrow). E and F, The leak was posterior and midline, measuring 4.6×5.6 mm in orthogonal views on the CT (arrows). A thick CT maximum intensity projection (MIP) image was then created to mimic fluoroscopy of the aortic valve prosthesis. G, The angle was identified on CT that visually placed the leak at the edge of the aortic valve prosthesis, superimposed for a single view (crosshairs). H, This angle was then reproduced in the cardiac catheterization laboratory for rapid wire crossing of the defect (arrow). I, A single 12-mm vascular plug type II (St. Jude Medical, St. Paul, MN) (arrow) was effective in treating the regurgitation, and the patient was discharged the following day.

AML, Anterior mitral leaflet; Ao, ascending aorta; AVR, aortic valve replacement; LA, left atrium; LV, left ventricle; RV, right ventricle.

KEY POINTS

- Cardiac CT angiography provides incremental diagnostic data to help identify an aortic paravalvular leak.
- Identification of the leak on CT allows determination of the fluoroscopic angle, which then facilitates crossing with a guidewire for percutaneous closure.
- Failure to identify a defect on CT should raise concern that the AI is not paravalvular.

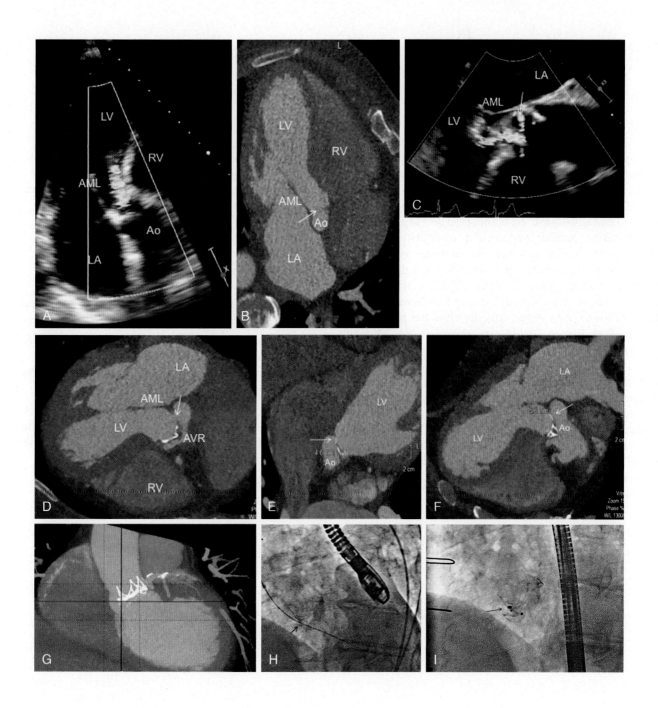

Retrograde Repair of Aortic Paravalvular Regurgitation

Paul Sorajja, MD

A 72-year-old woman with dyspnea is referred for percutaneous closure of aortic paravalvular regurgitation. She previously underwent aortic valve replacement with a 27-mm bi-leaflet mechanical prosthesis (St. Jude Medical, St. Paul, MN). Transesophageal echocardiography (TEE) demonstrates severe anterior paravalvular regurgitation (arrowheads) in (A) a long-axis and (B) short-axis view. C, An AL-1 diagnostic catheter, placed from the right femoral artery, is steered toward the defect, which is then crossed with a 260-cm, angle-tipped, extra-stiff Glidewire (arrowhead) (Terumo, Ann Arbor, MI). D, Over the glidewire, a 90-cm, 8-Fr Flexor Shuttle (arrowhead) (Cook Medical, Bloomington, IN) is passed into the left ventricle (LV), followed by placement of two 0.032″ extra-stiff Amplatz wires. Over these two wires, two separate 6-Fr Flexor Shuttle sheaths are advanced into the LV. The distal retention discs of two 10-mm Type II Amplatzer vascular plugs (St. Jude Medical, St. Paul, MN) are extruded in the LV, (E) followed by retraction and apposition against the left ventricular side and (F) deployed (arrowhead). The final view is chosen to demonstrate normal prosthetic leaflet motion. Postprocedural TEE in (G) long-axis and (H) short-axis views demonstrates mild residual regurgitation.

Ao, Ascending aorta; LA, left atrium; LV, left ventricle; RA, right atrium.

KEY POINTS

- The retrograde approach is preferred for percutaneous closure of an aortic paravalvular regurgitation.
- The use of multiple, relatively smaller device occluders minimizes the risk of leaflet impingement.
- Multiple delivery catheters can be placed simultaneously over separate extra-stiff Amplatz wires.
- A 12- to 24-Fr DrySeal sheath (W.L. Gore and Associates; Flagstaff, AZ) maintains vascular hemostasis when using simultaneous delivery catheters are needed.

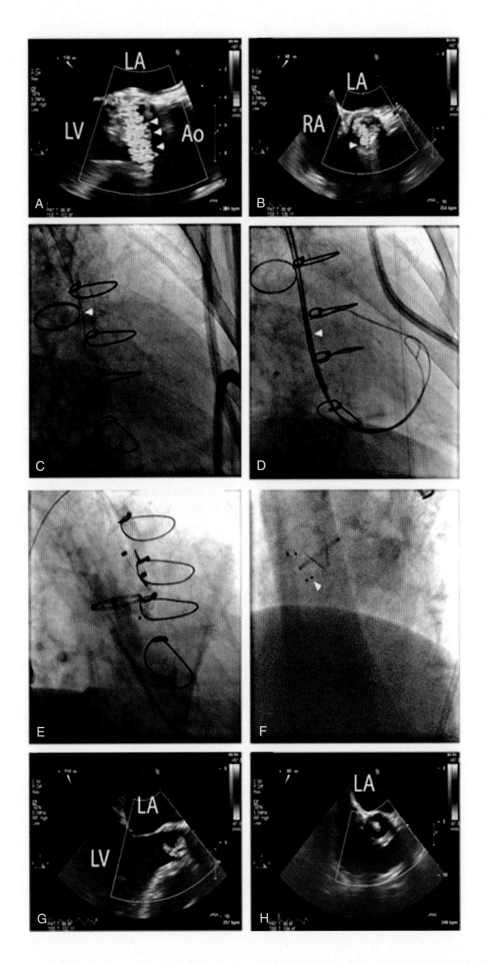

Retrograde Repair of Mitral Paravalvular Regurgitation for Recurrent Paravalvular Regurgitation

Tilak K. R. Pasala, MD, Vladimir Jelnin, MD, and Carlos E. Ruiz, MD, PhD

A 94-year-old woman presented with heart failure and hemolysis. She first underwent mitral valve (MV) repair 9 years ago, then had re-operation with MV replacement using a 25-mm Mosaic a year later. Two months ago, transseptal mitral paravalvular leak (PVL) closure was performed with two Type II Amplatzer vascular plugs (AVP) (St. Jude Medical, St. Paul, MN). A–D, Transesophageal echocardiography (TEE) showed recurrent severe PVL from the posterolateral aspect of the sewing ring. E, Fluoroscopy showed migration of a device toward the left ventricle (black arrow). Transapical access was obtained, and a 6-Fr 45-cm Terumo sheath (Terumo Corp., Tokyo, Japan) was advanced over a Neff wire (Cook Medical, Bloomington, IN) (white arrow) through the PVL lesion into the left atrium. The Neff wire was exchanged for a 35-cm Inoue wire (Toray Medical Co., Tokyo, Japan). F, Two 8-mm AVP II devices were advanced and positioned in the left atrium (white arrow). Subsequently, with simultaneous movements, the two AVPs were positioned across the leak until significant reduction in the PVL was noted on TEE. G, The Inoue wire was then removed, and the AVP II devices were sequentially released (white arrow). The 6-Fr sheath was slowly withdrawn to the left ventricular apex. The endocardial border was identified with a contrast injection through the side-arm. Anticoagulation was reversed at this point. H, A third 8-mm AVP II device was deployed in the apex and released after echocardiography demonstrated no pericardial effusion (white arrow). Floseal (Baxter Healthcare Corp., Deerfield IL) was then injected in the sheath as it was withdrawn, with manual pressure applied over the puncture site for hemostasis.

KEY POINTS

- Migration of the AVP II device may occur after percutaneous PVL closure.
- Percutaneous transapical access with fusion-imaging guidance facilitated closure with accuracy and precision, thereby lowering the risk of device embolization.
- Hemostasis of the left ventricular apex can be obtained with placement of AVP devices and Floseal.

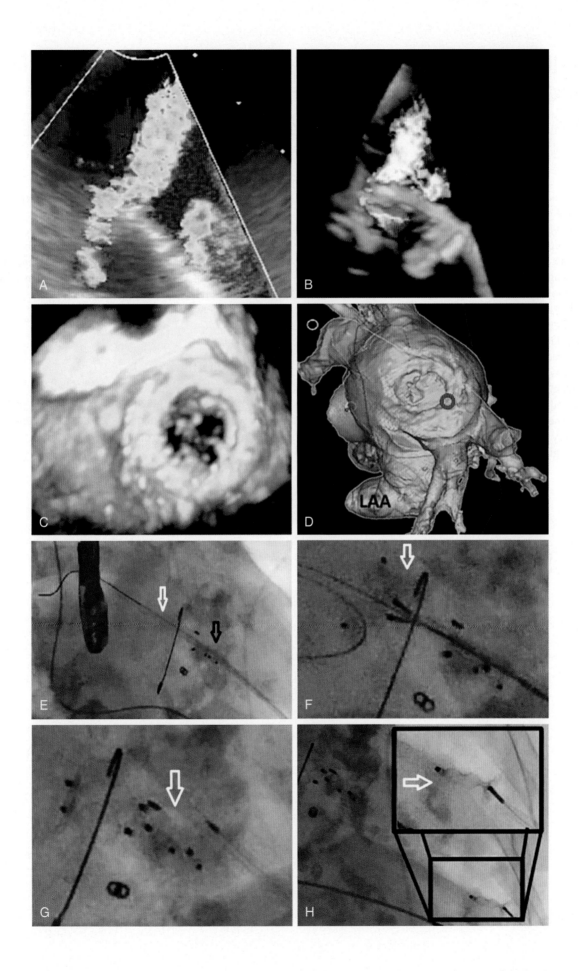

Retrograde Repair of a Multi-Orifice Mitral Paravalvular Leak by Hopscotch Technique

Tilak K. R. Pasala, MD, Vladimir Jelnin, MD, and Carlos E. Ruiz, MD, PhD

A 77-year-old man presented with progressive dyspnea and anemia, and was referred for percutaneous closure of severe mitral paravalvular leak (PVL). He had undergone mitral valve replacement with a #31 St. Jude mechanical prosthesis (St. Jude Medical, St. Paul, MN) 18 years ago. A and B, Transesophageal echocardiography (TEE) and 3-dimensional reconstruction using a cardiac computed tomography angiogram (CTA) demonstrated a severe multi-orifice PVL (white arrows). Two PVLs are seen separated by suture line in the posterolateral aspect of the valve. The Hopscotch technique is used to deliver multiple devices into consecutive PVLs. Transapical access was obtained. Then, PVL was crossed with a 6-Fr, 25-cm catheter over a glidewire, which is exchanged for an Inoue wire. C and D, A delivery catheter with the device is advanced, but is left attached (1). The delivery sheath is then pulled back to give enough distance for a glidewire to cross the adjacent PVL (3). Then the Inoue wire is pulled back and the device is deployed. This maneuver allows the delivery sheath to "hop" to the adjacent PVL. An Amplatzer vascular plug (AVP) II device (St. Jude Medical, St. Paul, MN) is seen deployed (2). These steps are repeated until all the PVLs are closed with devices. In this case, three AVP II devices were placed as seen in the post-procedure (E) CTA and (F) TEE.

KEY POINTS

- The Hopscotch technique is a useful technique when closing contiguous or adjacent paravalvular leaks in close proximity.

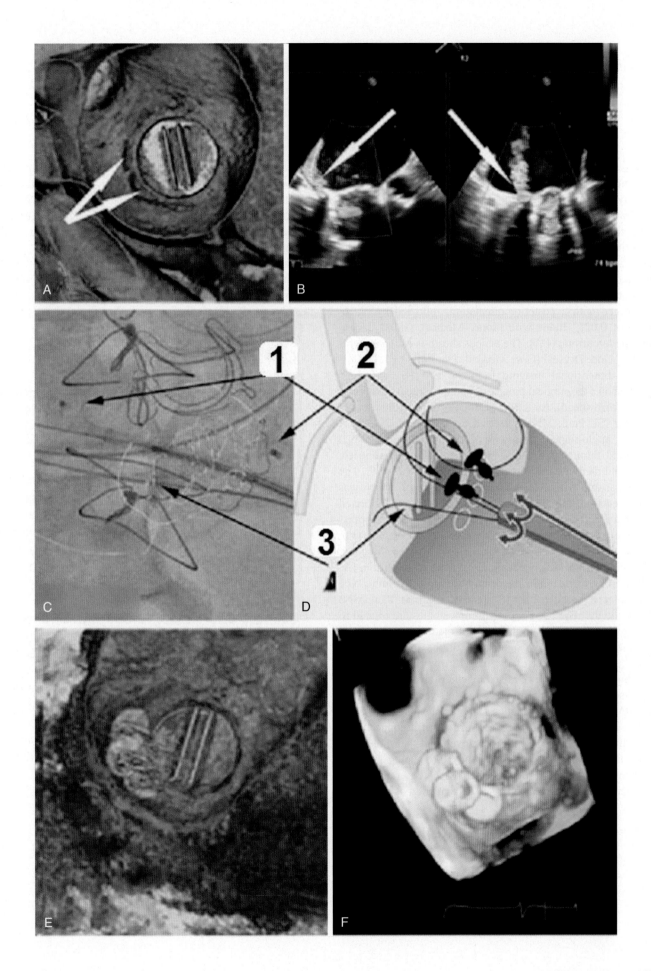

Antegrade Repair of Mitral Paravalvular Regurgitation

Paul Sorajja, MD

A 68-year-old woman presented with exertional dyspnea and evidence of severe paravalvular regurgitation involving a previously placed bileaflet, mechanical mitral prosthesis. A and B, Transesophageal echocardiography (TEE) demonstrates paravalvular regurgitation (arrowheads) arising medial to the mitral prosthesis (arrow) and anterior, close to the aortic valve annulus. Femoral venous access is obtained, followed by placement of 2 Proglide sutures in a preclose technique (Abbott Vascular, Santa Clara, CA). Transseptal puncture is performed with a posterior orientation, followed by placement of 0.025″ Inoue wire (Toray Medical, Chiba, Japan) into the left atrium (LA). The venous sheath is exchanged for a 20-Fr Gore Dryseal (Gore Medical, Flagstaff, AZ). C, TEE with 3-dimensional imaging from the LA (i.e., surgeon's view) shows the surgical prosthesis and the large paravalvular defect (arrowhead). An 8.5-Fr St. Jude Agilis, medium-curve catheter (St. Paul, MN) is steered toward the defect. D, A 0.035″ angle-tipped Glidewire (Terumo, Somerset, NJ) is passed through the defect (arrow) into the left ventricle (LV), and then into the descending aorta (arrowhead). E, The wire is snared with a 15-mm gooseneck (arrow), which was advanced from the left femoral artery, and then exteriorized to create a rail (arrow). F, This exteriorized rail both supports passage of delivery sheaths and serves as an anchor wire (AW). A 90-cm, 8-Fr Flexor Shuttle sheath (Cook Medical, Bloomington, IN) (S) is advanced over the wire into the LV, followed by extrusion of the distal portion of a 10-mm, type II Amplatzer Vascular Plug (St. Jude Medical, St. Paul, MN) alongside the wire. G, The fluoroscopic angles are rotated to an angle perpendicular to the plane of the mitral valve (MV) prosthesis to facilitate examination of the prosthetic leaflets during deployment of the plug (arrow). H, The vascular plug and sheath are retracted together (arrow) to position the distal portion of the plug on the left ventricular side of the MV prosthesis. I, The plug is then unsheathed across the defect (arrows). J, With the plug (arrows) still connected to its delivery cable, the sheath is removed and then reinserted over only the anchor wire. A second 10-mm plug (arrows) is then deployed in similar fashion. K, Once effectiveness has been established and there is no evidence of prosthetic

leaflet impingement, the anchor wire is removed. Both plugs (arrows) are then decoupled from their delivery catheters. Imaging with TEE in (L) commissural and (M) left ventricular outflow tract views shows minimal residual regurgitation (arrowheads). N, Final imaging with 3-dimensional TEE shows the two plugs in place (arrows).

Ant, Anterior; Ao, ascending aorta; AW, anchor wire; D, Delivery catheter; L, lateral; LA, left atrium; LV, left ventricle; M, medial; MV, mitral valve; S, Shuttle sheath, SGC, steerable guide catheter.

KEY POINTS

- Leaflet impingement is one of the most common modes of failure for percutaneous repair of paravalvular regurgitation. Use of multiple, relatively smaller plugs to minimize device overhang helps to avoid leaflet impingement in these cases.
- An exteriorized rail facilitates the procedure by serving as an anchor wire and supporting passage of delivery catheters. This rail is created with snaring of the soft portion of the wire from the contralateral femoral artery, and exteriorization through the sheath. With gentle tension on both ends of the rail, delivery catheters can be pulled across serpiginous and rigid defects.
- A large bore (i.e., 20-Fr Gore Dryseal) sheath accommodates multiple catheters and wires, including the rail and delivery cables. The balloon occlusion cuff helps with hemostasis.
- The 8-Fr Flexor Shuttle sheath allows passage of type II Amplatzer Vascular plugs up to 16 mm in diameter alongside a 0.035″ wire rail.
- The transseptal puncture should be posterior for medial defects to minimize angulation for steering and delivery catheter passage.

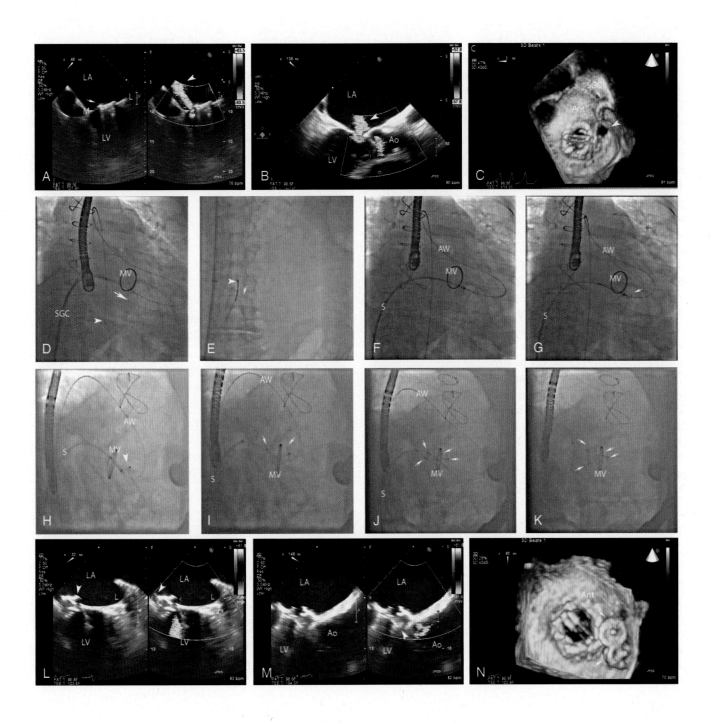

Benefit of Accurate Transseptal Puncture in Paravalvular Closure

Paul Sorajja, MD

A 73-year-old woman was referred for treatment of symptomatic mitral paravalvular regurgitation. Six years ago, she underwent cardiac surgery with placement of mechanical tilting disc prostheses in the aortic and mitral positions for severe rheumatic heart disease. The patient then developed debilitating exertional dyspnea. A, On transesophageal echocardiography (TEE), there was severe, medial paravalvular regurgitation (arrowhead). B, The initial transseptal puncture was superior and anterior. This location is seen on three-dimensional (3-D) TEE imaging, where a pre-shaped guidewire has been placed across the atrial septum (arrowhead). C, An 8.5-Fr Agilis, medium-curve catheter (St. Jude Medical, St. Paul, MN) is placed with telescoping 5-Fr and 6-Fr multipurpose catheters in the left atrium. A 0.035″, angle-tipped exchange-length Glidewire is passed into the defect (arrowhead) (Terumo, Somerset, NJ). D, Fluoroscopic imaging showing the guidewire (arrowhead) passing through the paravalvular defect into the left ventricle. However, because of the steep, superior-inferior trajectory from the transseptal puncture to the paravalvular defect, the multipurpose catheters (MP) could not be advanced across the defect. Creation of a rail was not pursued because the operator did not want to cross the mechanical aortic valve and also did not want to puncture the left ventricular apex. E, The transseptal puncture was repeated with a more posterior orientation (arrowhead). F and G, On 3-D TEE imaging, the location of the transseptal puncture (arrow) is confirmed to be relatively inferior and posterior, and there is more coaxial alignment of the steerable catheter (arrowheads) with the inferior site of the paravalvular defect. H and I, The second transseptal location enables easy crossing of the defect with the wire (arrow) and a 6-Fr multipurpose guide catheter (arrowhead), without the need for additional support. J and K, A 12-mm, Type II Amplatzer Vascular Plug (arrowheads) (St. Jude Medical, St. Paul, MN) is deployed across the defect with elimination of the paravalvular leak.

Ant, Anterior; Ao, ascending aorta; AV, aortic valve; IAS, interatrial septum; LA, left atrium; LV, left ventricle; MV, mitral valve; Post, posterior; RA, right atrium; SGC, steerable guide catheter.

KEY POINTS

- For many structural heart interventions, the location of the transseptal puncture is a "make-or-break" part of the procedure.
- The desired location depends on the specific interventional procedure, and should be obtained with guidance from either transesophageal or intracardiac echocardiography. 3-D imaging of the atrial septum can be helpful.
- A 6-Fr multipurpose guide catheter will accommodate a 12-mm Type II Amplatzer Vascular Plug.

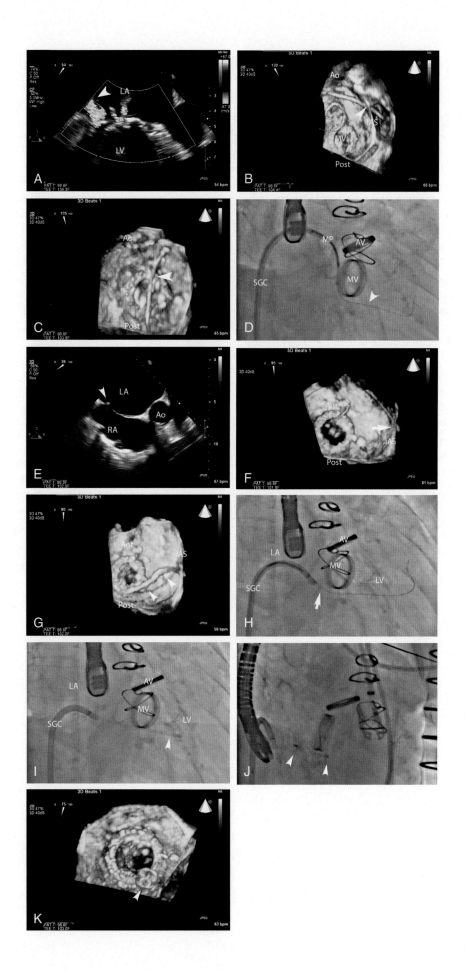

Challenging Echocardiographic Imaging for Paravalvular Leak Closure

Richard Y. Bae, MD

A 43-year-old man underwent mitral valve replacement with a 31-mm Hancock bioprosthesis 1 year ago at an outside institution, and was referred for severe paravalvular regurgitation. The patient suffered from significant symptoms of dyspnea and fatigue. A, Transesophageal echocardiography (TEE) revealed a severe paravalvular leak near the left atrial appendage orifice (arrow). B, On 3-dimensional (3-D) TEE imaging, there was a large arc of tissue dropout in this region (arrows). This tissue dropout on 3-D imaging can be misleading, and lead to overestimation of the size of the paravalvular defect. C, Flipping the image over to the perspective of the left ventricle, and using color Doppler can help better identify the extent of the regurgitant orifice (arrow). D, Transseptal puncture is performed under TEE guidance. E, The Agilis steerable catheter (St. Jude Medical, St. Paul, MN) is advanced to the region of defect, and a Glidewire is advanced into the defect (arrow). F, To visualize the wire entering the defect, the 3-D image will often need to be tilted to view the region of interest from a slightly more lateral perspective (arrow). G, After a 16-mm Type II Amplatzer vascular plug (AVP) (St. Jude Medical, St. Paul, MN) was deployed (arrow), (H) there was still significant paravalvular regurgitation (arrow). I, A total of three 16-mm AVP 2 plugs were deployed (arrow), (J) with trivial residual regurgitation at the end of the procedure (arrow). The mean diastolic gradient across the bioprosthesis actually fell from 8 mm Hg at baseline (K) to 5 mm Hg after paravalvular leak closure (L).

A, Anterior; Ao, ascending aorta; CS, coronary sinus; L, lateral; LA, left atrium; LV, left ventricle; M, medial; MV, mitral valve; P, posterior; RA, right atrium.

KEY POINTS

- Tissue dropout on 3-D imaging can lead to overestimation of the size of the paravalvular defect. Color imaging on 3-D from the ventricular aspect can facilitate more accurate sizing of the regurgitant orifice.
- For paravalvular leaks that originate directly underneath the sewing ring, tilting the 3-D image to view the defect from a relatively lateral perspective can be helpful.
- Complete assessment of procedural result includes determination of residual regurgitation, leaflet impingement, and mitral gradients.

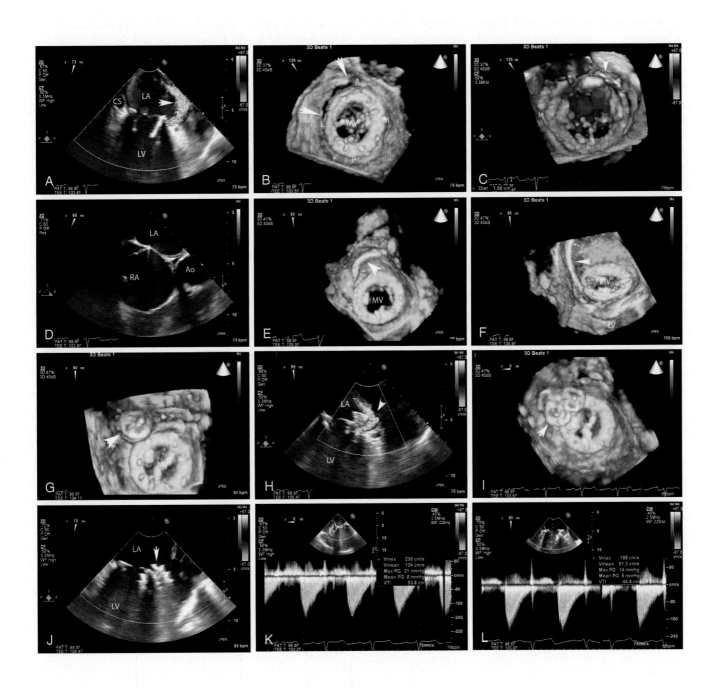

Coronary Dissection From Paravalvular Leak Closure

Paul Sorajja, MD

An 66-year-old man was referred for percutaneous treatment of paravalvular aortic regurgitation. He previously underwent placement of a 23-mm Epic bioprosthesis (St. Jude Medical, Fridley, MN), and had persistent, severe symptoms attributable to the paravalvular regurgitation. A, Parasternal, transthoracic echocardiography showing the aortic valve prosthesis (AV). The left ventricular function was normal. B, Doppler color-flow imaging shows anterior paravalvular regurgitation (arrow). C, A 6-Fr multipurpose catheter is used to pass an exchange-length, Glidewire (Terumo, Somerset, NJ) (arrowhead). D, The wire (arrowhead) passes easily into the left ventricle, then exits the aortic valve. E, The operator attempts to place a 90-cm, 8-Fr Flexor Shuttle sheath (Cook Medical, Bloomington, IN) (arrowhead) but is unsuccessful. While preparing to snare the wire to create a rail for more support, the patient begins to complain of chest pain. F, Coronary angiography demonstrates coronary dissection of both the left anterior descending artery (arrow) and the ramus intermedius artery (arrowhead). G, Emergent percutaneous coronary intervention with placement of multiple drug-eluting stents in these two vessels is performed. The left circumflex artery was previously grafted, and therefore not addressed percutaneously. H, Left anterior oblique view when the operator thought the Glidewire was across the paravalvular defect. Note the considerable distance of the wire from the aortic bioprosthesis and its trajectory over the lateral surface of the heart (arrowhead). These features indicate the wire was actually down the ramus intermedius artery. Six weeks later, the patient returned for percutaneous repair of the paravalvular regurgitation, with successful placement of a single, 12-mm Type II Amplatzer Vascular Plug (St. Jude Medical, Fridley, MN).

Ao, Ascending aorta; AV, aortic valve; MP, multipurpose; LA, left artery; LV, left ventricle; RV, right ventricle.

KEY POINTS

- When performing percutaneous repair of aortic paravalvular regurgitation, the guidewire can easily be placed into the coronary arteries. Confirmation of path of the wire on both fluoroscopy and echocardiography are essential for procedure success.
- When there is concern for placement of the guidewire in the coronary artery, fluoroscopy in the left anterior oblique view is useful.

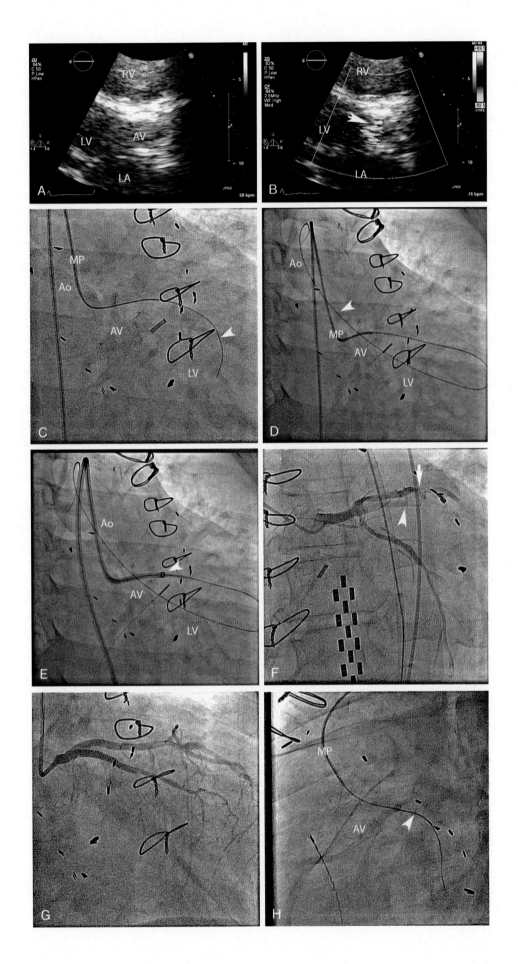

Treatment of Coronary Obstruction After Paravalvular Leak Closure

Hussam S. Suradi, MD, and Samer Abbas, MD

An 80-year-old man presented with chest pain two years after successful paravalvular aortic leak closure. The patient previously underwent surgical aortic valve replacement with a 23-mm bioprosthetic valve, complicated by severe paravalvular leak originating close to the left coronary cusp that resulted in symptomatic heart failure. He underwent successful paravalvular leak closure using a 6-mm Amplatzer Duct Occluder II (ADO II) device (St. Jude Medical, Plymouth, MN) with complete resolution of the leak and symptomatic improvement. Ascending aortography was performed at the end of the procedure that showed adequate opacification of both coronary arteries at that time. Two years later, the patient presented with exertional chest pain. Echocardiography showed normal prosthetic aortic valve function and no evidence of paravalvular leak. A, Selective coronary angiography suggested the possibility of partial obstruction of the left main ostium by the proximal disk of the ADO II device (arrow). B, This obstruction was confirmed by intravascular ultrasound, with minimal luminal area of 4.23 mm^2 at the ostium of the left main artery (asterisk denotes the proximal disk of the ADO II). A 4.0- × 8-mm Synergy drug-eluting stent (Boston Scientific, Natick, MA) was implanted within the left main ostium extending just proximal to the disk of the occluder device (C), and was postdilated with a 5.0-mm noncompliant balloon (D). Post-stenting angiogram (E) and intravascular ultrasound (F, asterisk denotes the proximal disk of the ADO II) demonstrated exclusion of the occluder device and good expansion of the stent within the left main. The patient was discharged home with complete resolution of symptoms upon follow up.

KEY POINTS

- Operators must be aware of the possibility of obstruction of the left main ostium by the occluder with aortic paravalvular leak closure.
- In the setting of paravalvular leak closure close to the left coronary cusp, selective coronary angiography in multiple projections is recommended to identify possible left main obstruction, with device retrieval if indicated.
- Intravascular ultrasound-guided stent implantation is a feasible approach for the treatment of left main impingement that is identified after occluder device release.

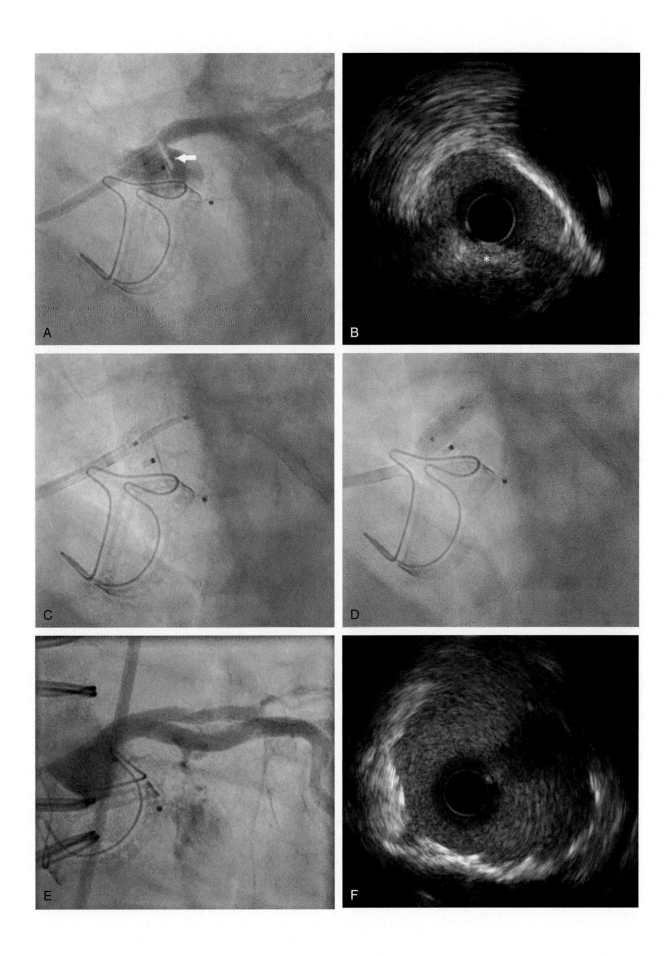

Papillary Muscle Rupture During Paravalvular Leak Closure

Paul Sorajja, MD

A 77-year-old man was referred for treatment of symptomatic aortic paravalvular regurgitation involving a 25-mm Trifecta tissue prosthesis (St. Jude Medical, Fridley, MN). A, Short-axis view of the aortic valve prosthesis on transesophageal echocardiography (TEE) demonstrates paravalvular regurgitation involving the left cusp (arrowhead). B, On a long-axis, TEE view, the aortic paravalvular regurgitation is noted to be severe (arrowhead). C, The paravalvular defect is crossed with a 260-cm, 0.035″, angle-tipped exchange-length Glidewire (W, Terumo, Somerset, NJ), and a 6-Fr, 90-cm Cook Flexor catheter (C) is inserted. The arrow shows the direction of the wire passing into the left ventricle, followed by its passing through the aortic valve, where a 15-mm gooseneck snare has been positioned (arrowhead). D, The glidewire is snared and exteriorized (arrowhead) out the contralateral femoral artery. Tension is then applied to both ends of the wire to pull the Flexor catheter across the paravalvular defect. E–G, On multiple views using TEE, rupture of the papillary muscle head is evident (arrowheads). H, On color-compare TEE imaging, new, severe eccentric mitral regurgitation is present in association with the papillary muscle rupture (arrowhead). I, Specimen of the ruptured papillary muscle obtained when the patient went to cardiac surgery for mitral valve (MV) replacement.

Ao, Ascending aorta; AV, aortic valve prosthesis; C, Cook flexor catheter; LA, left atrium; LV, left ventricle; Post, posterior; RV, right ventricle; W, Glidewire.

KEY POINTS

- For the percutaneous treatment of aortic paravalvular regurgitation, creation of an aortic-arterial rail provides significant support for placement of delivery catheters.
- When placing these aorta-arterial rails, one must be careful not to entangle the MV apparatus. A meticulous echocardiographic evaluation of the MV during placement of the rail and while applying tension is essential to the successful use of this technique.

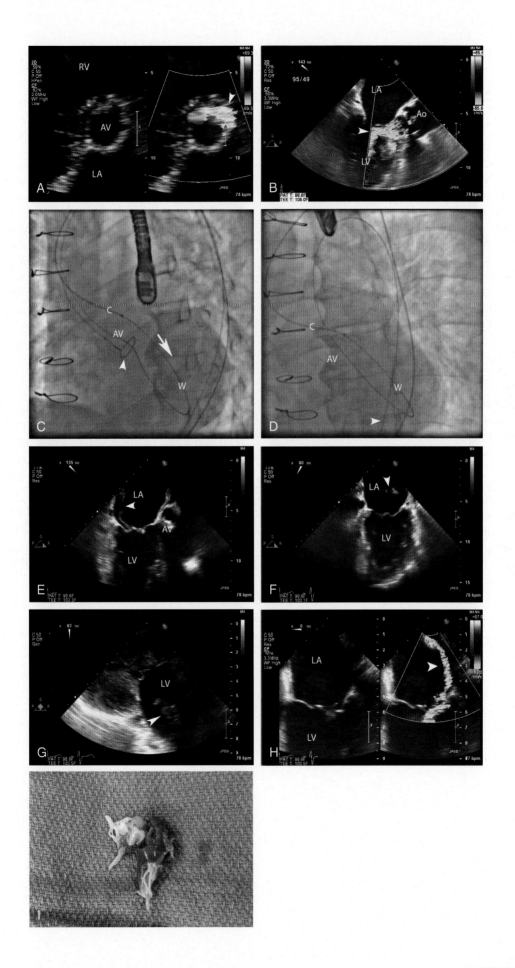

Step-up Technique With Aortic Paravalvular Leak Closure

Paul Sorajja, MD

An 80-year-old man, who was previously treated with transcatheter aortic valve replacement using a 31-mm CoreValve prosthesis (Medtronic, Dublin, Ireland), was referred for percutaneous therapy of symptomatic aortic paravalvular regurgitation. A, Using a retrograde approach from the right femoral artery, a 6-Fr AL-1 diagnostic catheter was placed above the defect, which was posterolateral to the aortic prosthesis. Initially, an angle-tipped Glidewire (Terumo, Ann Arbor, MI) was employed to attempt to cross the defect. However, the stiffness of the wire changed the direction of the coronary catheter during any advancement of the wire, reducing precision for steering to the defect. The defect was then wired successfully with a soft 0.014″, 300-cm Whisper coronary guidewire (Abbott Vascular, Santa Clara, CA) (arrowheads). B, A 2.3-Fr QuickCross catheter (arrows; Spectranetics, Colorado Springs, CO) was used to exchange for a 0.018″ Glidewire (arrowhead), which advanced into the aorta. C, A 6-Fr Flexor Shuttle (Cook Medical, Bloomington, IN) (DC; arrow) was advanced to the defect, but could not be passed into the left ventricle. The Glidewire was then snared with a gooseneck in the ascending aorta (arrowhead). D, With tension on the wire (arrowhead), the delivery catheter (arrow) was easily pulled across the defect and into the left ventricle. E, A 6-mm Type II Amplatzer vascular plug (arrow; St. Jude Medical, St. Paul, MN) was advanced with the 0.018″ Glidewire (arrowhead) remaining to serve as a rail and an anchor wire. F, The plug is straddled across the defect (arrows). G, With the plug still attached (arrowhead), contrast injection through the Flexor shuttle is performed to demonstrate no interference with the left coronary artery. H, The plug (arrowheads) is decoupled from the delivery cable. I, Preprocedural transthoracic echocardiography demonstrates significant paravalvular regurgitation (arrowhead). J, Following treatment, transesophageal echocardiography with color-compare imaging demonstrates no residual regurgitation (arrow) with the plug in place (arrowhead).

DC, Delivery catheter; LA, left atrium; LCA, left coronary artery; LV, left ventricle; MCV, Medtronic CoreValve.

KEY POINTS

- When performing retrograde repair of aortic paravalvular regurgitation, stiffness with relatively large wires (for example, 0.035″) can reduce fidelity of positioning, and prolong or inhibit successful cannulation. The use of soft, coronary guidewires can overcome this challenge.

- To facilitate snaring and creation of a rail, the coronary guidewire can be exchanged for a larger wire using exchange catheters, such as the QuickCross catheter, which accommodates 0.018″ wires.

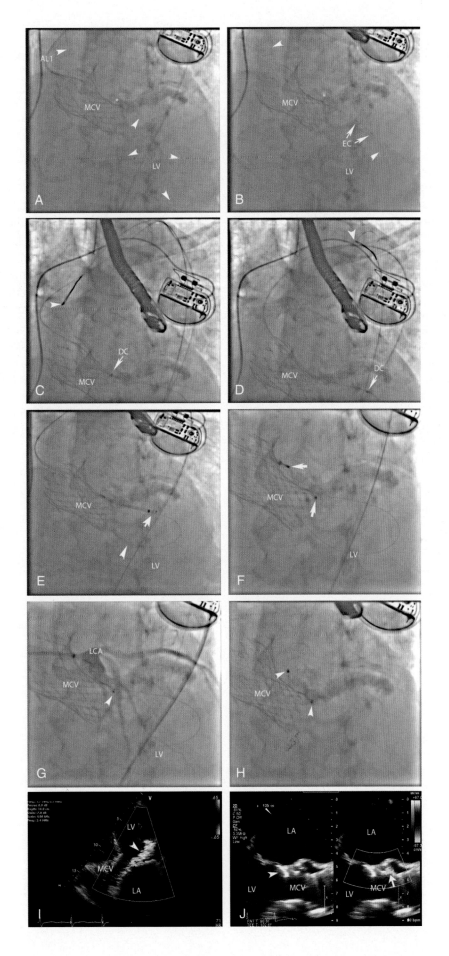

The Anchor Wire Technique for Aortic Paravalvular Leak Closure

Paul Sorajja, MD

A 55-year-old man was referred for percutaneous closure of aortic paravalvular regurgitation. The patient previously underwent cardiac surgery with placement of bi-leaflet mechanical prostheses (St. Jude Medical, St. Paul, MN) in both the aortic and mitral positions. A and B, At baseline, transthoracic echocardiography shows severe paravalvular regurgitation in multiple apical long-axis views (arrowheads). C, The paravalvular defect was crossed using a 6-Fr multipurpose catheter and a 260-cm, angle-tipped, extra-stiff Glidewire (arrow) (Terumo, Ann Arbor, MI). Care was taken to ensure the wire passed through the paravalvular defect external to the mechanical aortic valve prosthesis (arrowheads, C and D). E, The glidewire was passed antegrade through the mechanical aortic valve safely (arrow) to provide adequate support for passage of a 6-Fr Flexor Shuttle sheath into the left ventricle (arrowhead) (Cook Medical, Bloomington, IN). F, A 0.032″ extra-stiff Amplatz wire is inserted (arrowhead). G, A 12-mm Type II Amplatzer vascular plug (arrowhead) is positioned across the paravalvular defect with the Amplatz wire (arrow) remaining in the left ventricle, followed by ascending aortography. H, Final image after decoupling of the plug (arrow) from the delivery cable. Repeat fluoroscopy to document normal leaflet motion is performed.

Ao, Ascending aorta; LA, left atrium; LV, left ventricle.

KEY POINTS

- For patients undergoing percutaneous closure of aortic paravalvular regurgitation, the use of an anchor wire saves procedure time by reducing the need to re-cross the defect in the event additional or different occluders are required. A 6-Fr Flexor sheath will accommodate both a 12-mm AVP-2 plug and 0.032″ extra-stiff Amplatz wire.
- Prior to release of the device occluder, aortography is performed to confirm relief of regurgitation and demonstrate patency of the coronary arteries, which may arise near the treated paravalvular defects.
- Recording of normal leaflet motion is important to demonstrate no leaflet impingement with occluder placement.

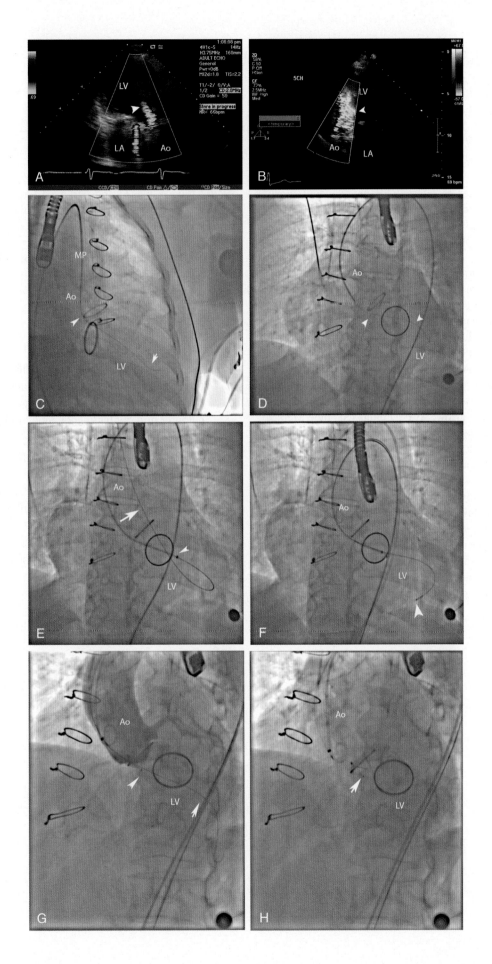

Rewiring in Sequential Plug Placement for Paravalvular Regurgitation

Paul Sorajja, MD

A 74-year-old woman is referred for percutaneous closure of mitral paravalvular regurgitation involving a 27-mm bi-leaflet mechanical prosthesis (St. Jude Medical, St. Paul, MN). A, Transesophageal echocardiography (TEE) with color flow imaging demonstrates severe mitral paravalvular regurgitation (arrowhead). B, TEE with 3-dimensional (3-D) imaging from the left atrium (i.e., surgeon's view) shows a large dehiscence in the lateral aspect of the mitral prosthesis (arrowheads). C, Following transseptal puncture, the defect is crossed with a 260-cm, angle-tipped, extra-stiff Glidewire (arrow) (Terumo, Ann Arbor, MI) placed from an 8.5-Fr steerable Agilis catheter (SGC, St. Jude Medical, St. Paul, MN). The wire is passed antegrade and snared in the descending aorta (arrowhead). D, Two 8-mm Type II Amplatzer vascular (arrow; AVP-2) plugs (St. Jude Medical, St. Paul, MN) are placed using sequential 6-Fr delivery catheters (90-cm Flexor Shuttle, Cook Medical, Bloomington, IN) with the glidewire serving as a rail. E, These occluders are visible on TEE with 3-D imaging (arrows). F, However, severe mitral paravalvular regurgitation persists (arrowhead). G, The origin of this regurgitation is superior to the previously placed plugs (arrow). Additional devices cannot be placed in the target area due to relatively fixed positioning of the rail. H, The rail is removed and the defect is rewired with the glidewire using the Agilis catheter, and crossed with a 6-Fr multipurpose catheter (arrow). I and J, A third, 8-mm AVP-2 plug is placed and deployed (arrows). K, TEE with 3-D imaging shows the three plugs in place (arrow). L, Following implantation, the residual mitral regurgitation is mild (arrow).

LA, Left atrium; LV, left ventricle; MV, mitral valve; SGC, steerable guide catheter.

KEY POINTS

- Use of a veno-arterial rail facilitates percutaneous treatment of mitral paravalvular regurgitation, by providing support for passage of the delivery catheter and enabling sequential, multiple catheter placement.
- However, the rail may become relatively fixed in position and not allow targeting of areas of residual regurgitation. In these instances, the rail may need to be removed, followed by rewiring of the defect with a steerable catheter.
- Each of the device occluders remains connected to their delivery cables until final deployment, to reduce the risk of embolization.

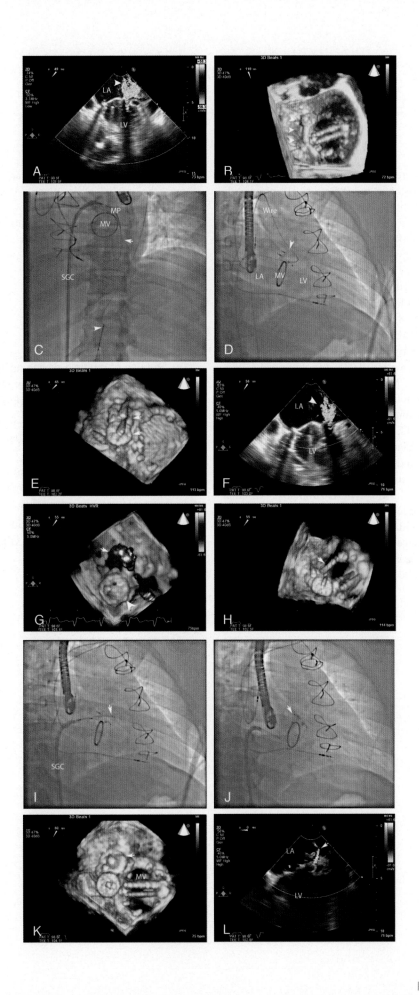

Simultaneous Plug Placement for Paravalvular Leaks

Paul Sorajja, MD

A 78-year-old was referred for percutaneous treatment of severe, paravalvular prosthetic regurgitation. He previously underwent surgery with placement of a 31-mm Hancock II prosthesis in the mitral position. A, Transesophageal echocardiography (TEE) demonstrates a large, medial defect with paravalvular regurgitation (arrowhead). B, The defect arose immediately inferior to the native aortic valve annulus (arrowhead). C, TEE with 3-dimensional (3-D) imaging shows medial paravalvular defect (arrow). D, Following transseptal puncture, an 8.5-Fr Agilis catheter (arrowhead) (St. Jude Medical, St. Paul, MN) is steered toward the defect using guidance from fluoroscopy and 3-D echocardiography. E, The defect is crossed with a 0.035″, angle-tipped Glidewire (Terumo, Somerset, NJ), which is passed through the defect into the left ventricle (LV). F, A telescoped 6-Fr multipurpose (MP) guide catheter is advanced into the LV over the guidewire (arrow). G, Two 0.032″ extra-stiff Amplatz wires (arrowheads) are placed through the MP catheter. The steerable Agilis is removed, followed by advancement of two separate 6-Fr, 90-cm Flexor Shuttle sheaths (Cook Medical, Bloomington, IN). H, A 12-mm type II Amplatzer Vascular Plug (arrowheads; St. Jude Medical, St. Paul, MN) is placed in each Flexor sheath with the 0.032″ wire left in place for anchoring. I, Both device occluders (arrow) are retracted to straddle the defect with retention disks on both sides. J, Both occluders are then decoupled from their delivery cables (arrows). K, TEE with 3-D imaging from the left atrial view shows the occluders in place (arrowhead). L, Following placement of the occluders (arrow), there is only a trivial degree of residual mitral regurgitation (arrowhead).

Ao, Aorta; L, lateral; LA, left atrium; LV, left ventricle; M, medial; MP, multipurpose; SG, steerable guide catheter.

KEY POINTS

- The use of multiple device occluders with relatively smaller size is helpful to reduce the risk of leaflet impingement and treat eccentric defects.
- These multiple occluders can be placed either sequentially or simultaneously, as shown in this case.
- The anchor wire saves procedural time by reducing the need to rewire the defect should additional or different occluders be needed.
- A 20-Fr DrySeal sheath (Gore Medical, Flagstaff, AZ) facilitates hemostasis when multiple delivery sheaths are utilized.

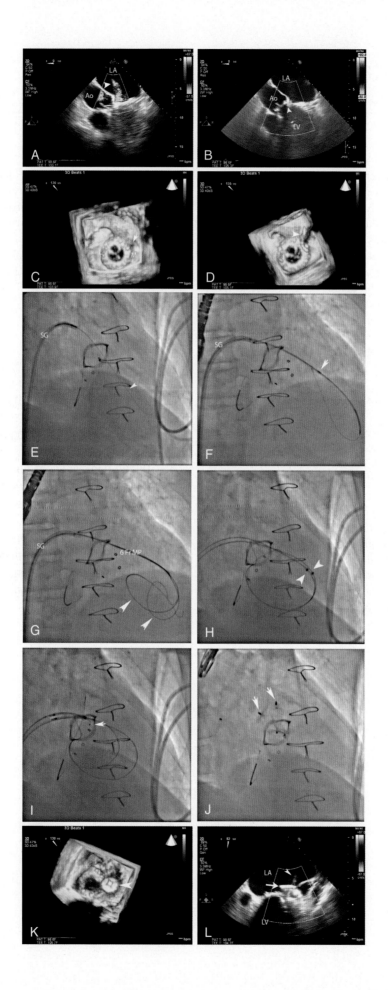

Closure of Aorta to Right Ventricle Fistula

Paul Sorajja, MD, Marcus Burns, DNP, and Judah Askew, MD

A 27-year-old man underwent urgent aortic valve replacement with a 23-mm On-X (CryoLife Inc., Kennesaw, GA) in the setting of prior aortic valve surgery for bicuspid disease. Shortly after surgery, a fistula from the noncoronary cusp to the right ventricle (RV) was evident on echocardiography, and the patient was brought to the cardiac catheterization laboratory for percutaneous closure. A, Short-axis transthoracic echocardiography of the aortic valve prosthesis (AV) demonstrates a fistula (arrowhead) arising from the noncoronary cusp. B, Apical 4-chamber view shows communication of this fistula (arrow) with the RV. C, Aortography of the ascending aorta confirms the presence of this fistula (arrow) draining into the RV (arrowheads). D, Using a 6-Fr multipurpose guide with a 5-Fr telescoped multipurpose catheter, the fistula was crossed with a 260-cm Glidewire (arrow) (Terumo, Somerset, NJ). E, Next, the 6-Fr multipurpose guide was advanced into the RV. F, The distal disc of a 12-mm Type II Amplatzer vascular plug (St. Jude Medical, St. Paul, MN) was extruded, but the initial position was too deep in the RV and the occluder was entangled in the tricuspid valve apparatus (arrowhead). G, The plug was gently re-sheathed, and then extruded closer to the base of the heart (direction of arrow), where there was no valvular entanglement (arrowhead). H, The plug is fully extruded (arrows), and fluoroscopy is performed to confirm no leaflet impingement. I, Aortography is performed to confirm occlusion of the fistula, as well as no interaction of the occluder (arrow) with coronary arteries. J, Final position of the occluder (arrow) following decoupling from the delivery cable. K, Short-axis transthoracic echocardiography showing position of the occluder after final release (arrow). L, Doppler color-flow imaging showing elimination of the regurgitation with the occluder in place (arrow).

Ao, Ascending aorta; AV, aortic valve prosthesis; LV, left ventricle; MP, multipurpose; RA, right atrium; RV, right ventricle.

KEY POINTS

- The approach to closure of fistulas from the aorta to the RV is similar to that used for closure of aortic paravalvular prosthetic regurgitation, and primarily entails the use of a retrograde approach with telescoping catheters.
- During deployment of the occluder in the RV, care must be undertaken to avoid entanglement with the tricuspid valve apparatus. Extrusion of the occluder at the base of the heart or close to the ventricular side of the defect may be required.
- As with all aortic interventions, the operator should be certain there is no leaflet impingement, and no interaction with the coronary ostia.

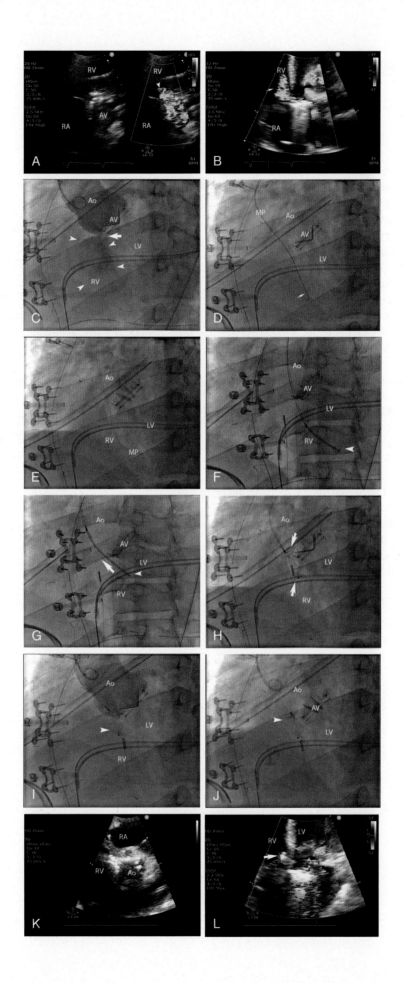

The Aortic Arterial Rail Technique

Paul Sorajja, MD

An 83-year-old man, who previously underwent transcatheter aortic valve replacement with a 26-mm Sapien S3 (Edwards Lifesciences, Irvine, CA), returned for persistent dyspnea in the setting of aortic paravalvular regurgitation. A, The paravalvular defect was crossed retrograde with a 0.014″, 300-cm Whisper coronary guidewire (arrowhead; Abbott Vascular, Santa Clara, CA) and an AL-1 diagnostic coronary catheter. B, The coronary wire (arrowhead; W) was passed antegrade to the ascending aorta. C, A 2.3-Fr Quickcross catheter (Spectranetics, Colorado Springs, CO) is advanced into the left ventricle (LV), followed by exchange for a 0.018″ Glidewire (Terumo, Ann Arbor, MI). The Glidewire is snared in the ascending aorta with a 15-mm gooseneck (arrow). D, With guidance from transesophageal echocardiography, tension is applied to both ends of the wire while ensuring there is no mitral valve (MV) entanglement. The wire is pulled (arrowheads) against the paravalvular defect and the Sapien valve (S). E, A 90-cm, 4-Fr Flexor Shuttle (arrows; Cook Medical, Bloomington, IN) is advanced through the defect and passes easily out of the aortic valve prosthesis (arrows). F, The sheath is retracted into the LV to avoid interaction of the occluder with aortic prosthetic leaflets during deployment. G, The distal disc of a 6-mm Type II Amplatzer vascular plug (AVP-2) (St. Jude Medical, St. Paul, MN) is placed in the LV (arrow), and then retracted and deployed across the paravalvular defect. H, Final imaging shows the AVP-2 plug deployed (arrows).

Ao, Ascending aorta; LV, left ventricle; S, Sapien S3 prosthesis; W, coronary guidewire.

KEY POINTS

- When performing percutaneous closure of aortic paravalvular regurgitation, creation of an aortic-arterial rail provides support for passage of delivery sheaths.
- Potential complications of this technique include entanglement of the rail with the MV apparatus, conduction abnormalities, and injury to the aortic prosthetic leaflets.
- The delivery sheath may cross the aortic valve prosthesis antegrade when the rail is created. In these instances, the distal portion of the delivery sheath should be positioned in the LV prior to placement of occluder to minimize interaction with the leaflets during deployment (e.g., impingement).

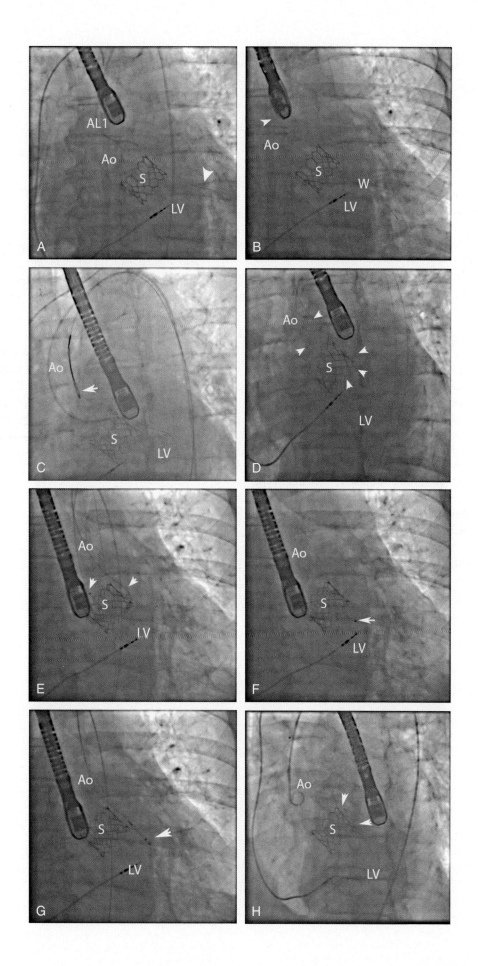

Repair of Paravalvular Regurgitation in a Balloon-Expanding Prosthesis

Paul Sorajja, MD

An 84-year-old man is referred for percutaneous closure of symptomatic aortic paravalvular regurgitation. Six months ago, he underwent successful transfemoral, transcatheter aortic valve replacement with a 26-mm Sapien XT (Edwards Lifesciences, Irvine, CA). He continued to have residual symptoms of lifestyle-limiting dyspnea. Paravalvular regurgitation involving transcatheter valves can be challenging to treat percutaneously, due to the need for navigation between the prosthesis and the intact native valve leaflets. Computed tomography (CT) with contrast can facilitate the success of such procedures. A, CT with contrast demonstrates a paravalvular defect in the posterior/superior aspect of the Sapien valve (arrows). The structures are aligned with a view of the defect immediately exterior and parallel to the valve prosthesis. B, These CT angles are provided to the operator, who places the image intensifier in the cardiac catheterization laboratory in the same position. C, With this positioning, the operator only has to pass the wire immediately exterior to the prosthesis (arrows). D, A 12-mm Amplatzer Vascular Type II Plug (St. Jude Medical, St. Paul, MN) is placed (arrow). Transesophageal echocardiography demonstrates the paravalvular leak (PVL) (E) before (arrow), and (F) after closure (arrow).

Ao, Aorta; LA, left atrium; LV, left ventricle.

KEY POINTS

- Percutaneous treatment of PVL involving transcatheter valves can be challenging as the guidewire must be navigated between the prosthesis and native leaflets.
- To facilitate the procedure, gated cardiac CT with contrast can be used to identify the site of the PVL, and provide data on its course and surrounding anatomy (for example, degree of calcification).
- Cardiac CT provides the angles for camera set-up for closure in the catheterization laboratory, allowing the operator to focus on passing the wire and delivery catheters immediately external to the prosthesis.

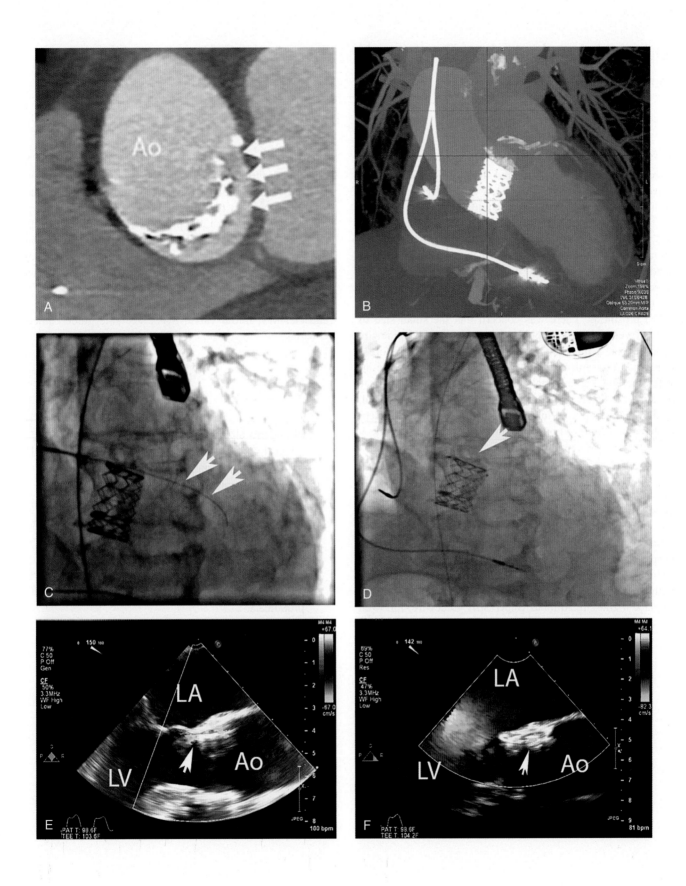

Mitral Valve-in-Valve Therapy With an Apical Rail

Paul Sorajja, MD

A 77-year-old woman with a recent history of decompensated heart failure was referred for transcatheter mitral valve replacement. Seven years ago, she underwent surgery with placement of a 29-mm St. Jude Epic mitral prosthesis for rheumatic mitral stenosis. A, Apical long-axis view on transthoracic echocardiography demonstrates severe mitral regurgitation (MR) on color-flow imaging (arrowhead). B, Transesophageal echocardiography (TEE) with three-dimensional imaging from the left atrium (LA) prior to the transcatheter therapy shows the degenerated mitral valve (MV) prosthesis. There was concern that the small size of her left ventricle (LV) would not permit enough guidewire support with a transseptal antegrade approach. Therefore a retrograde transapical approach to perform mitral valve-in-valve therapy was undertaken. C, An 8.5-Fr, medium-curve St. Jude Agilis steerable catheter (SGC) (St. Jude Medical, Fridley, MN) is placed in the LA using a posterior transseptal puncture, followed by positioning of a 15-mm gooseneck snare (arrowhead). With a surgical cut-down to the LV apex (Ap), a 6-Fr sheath (arrow) is placed into the LV through a transapical puncture. D, A 260-cm, angle-tipped Glidewire (Terumo) is passed from the 6-Fr sheath and across the MV prosthesis into the LA, where it is snared and exteriorized out the femoral vein (arrow). E, A 100-cm, 6-Fr multipurpose catheter is advanced retrograde and exteriorized (arrowheads) through the SGC. Note the central positioning of the catheter assembly across the MV that was made possible with steering of the SGC. The multipurpose catheter is used to place a 260-cm, Amplatz Super Stiff guidewire, followed by retrograde placement of an Ascendra transapical sheath (Edwards Lifesciences, Irvine, CA). F, A 29-mm Sapien XT is deployed during rapid ventricular pacing, with two-thirds of the prosthesis in the LV (S). Note that the SGC is retracted and there is support for positioning with the rail in place. G, Over the stiff wire (W), the prosthesis is postdilated to flare the LV portion (arrowheads). H, Final positioning of the new mitral prosthesis on fluoroscopy after wire removal. I, Postprocedural TEE shows trivial MR (arrowhead). J, The mean mitral gradient after implantation is only 2 mm Hg.

Ao, Ascending aorta; Ap, apex; LA, left atrium; LV, left ventricle; MV, mitral valve; SGC, steerable guide catheter; W, wire.

KEY POINTS

- When the size of the LV raises concern for wire support and prosthesis positioning, a transapical approach with creation of a veno-apical rail facilitates mitral valve-in-valve therapy.
- A steerable catheter in the LA facilitates central positioning of the guidewire across the prior surgical prosthesis, thereby enabling accurate positioning of the new mitral prosthesis.
- Flaring of the ventricular portion with postdilatation enhances stability of the newly placed mitral prosthesis.

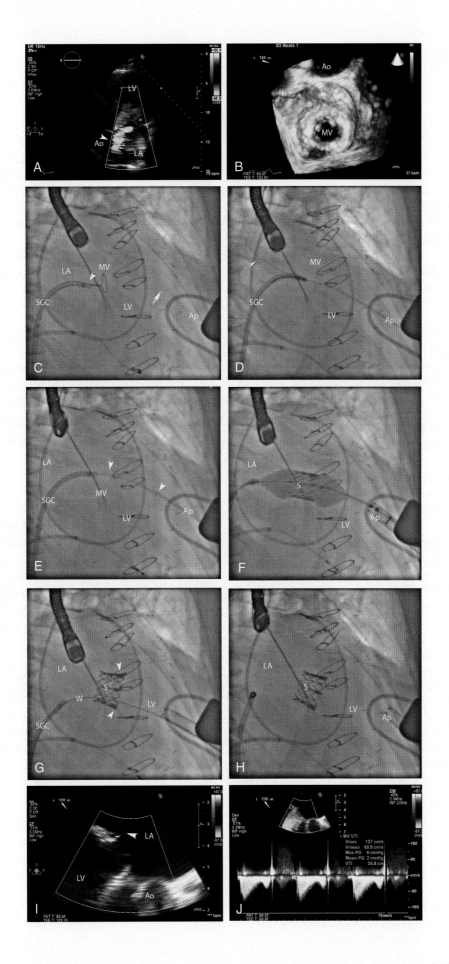

Antegrade Mitral Valve-in-Valve Therapy

Paul Sorajja, MD

An 82-year-old man presented for treatment of symptomatic, severe stenosis of a degenerated mitral prosthesis. Nine years ago, he underwent mitral surgery with placement of a 29-mm Edwards Magna prosthesis (Edwards Lifesciences, Irvine, CA), as well as surgical aortic valve replacement with a bioprosthesis. A transthoracic echocardiogram showed normal left ventricular function and severe stenosis with mean gradient of 12 mm Hg at a heart rate of 62 beats/min on Doppler imaging. A, End-diastolic image from transesophageal echocardiography (TEE) with 3-dimensional (3-D) imaging from the left atrium (LA) (i.e., surgeon's view) shows a degenerated mitral valve (MV) prosthesis with severe stenosis. B, On TEE, care is taken to perform the transseptal puncture with a posterior orientation (arrow), thereby minimizing the flexion needed to turn past the septum to the MV with the delivery catheter. C, An 8.5-Fr, medium-curve St. Jude Agilis steerable catheter (St. Jude Medical, Fridley, MN) is placed in the LA, and directed toward the MV prosthesis. D, A balloon wedge catheter (arrow) is floated from the LA into the left ventricle (LV). E, An extra-small curve Safari-2, pre-shaped guide wire (Boston Scientific, Maple Grove, MN) is placed in the LV (arrow), followed by alignment of the coaxial plane of the MV prosthesis on fluoroscopy (arrowhead). F and G, An 18-mm True balloon (arrowhead) (Bard Peripheral Vascular, Tempe, AZ) is used to gently dilate the septum with partial inflation and then the MV prosthesis is advanced over the Safari-2 guidewire (arrows). H, A 29-mm Sapien S3 (Edwards Lifesciences, Irvine, CA) is assembled on the delivery balloon in the inferior vena cava (arrowhead), followed by flexion and advancement to the MV prosthesis. I, The marker of the S3 prosthesis (arrowhead) is placed on the surgical valve, recognizing that shortening of the S3 will occur in the ventricular direction, and deployed with rapid ventricular pacing. The S3 prosthesis is not coaxial, but one can see the entire atrial portion located on in the LA. J, Final positioning shows the atrial portion of the S3 on the atrial side of the surgical prosthesis (arrowhead) with flaring of the ventricular portion to facilitate a cork-like anchoring effect. K, En face viewing of MV prosthesis in place (arrowhead). The atrial septum is closed with a 32-mm Amplatzer

Septal Occluder (ASO, St. Jude Medical, Fridley, MN). L, End-diastolic image on TEE with 3-D imaging showing full opening of the newly placed S3 prosthesis. (M) The final gradient across the newly placed S3 prosthesis was only 3 mm Hg, and (N) there was no evidence of mitral regurgitation on color-flow imaging with TEE.

Ao, Ascending aorta; LA, left atrium; LV, left ventricle; MV, mitral valve; RA, right atrium; SGC, steerable guide catheter.

KEY POINTS

- For mitral valve-in-valve therapy, the transseptal puncture should be posterior to gain height to the MV and thereby minimize the acuity of the angle toward the LV. Balloon dilatation of the atrial septum can help with antegrade passage of the prosthesis.
- A steerable, braided catheter can help to cross a stenotic mitral prosthesis and, with support from the articulation, facilitate placement of a stiff guidewire for the procedure. The balloon wedge catheter accommodates a 0.035″ guidewire.
- A preshaped guidewire placed in the LV suffices when the stiff segment is well across the mitral prosthesis and into the LV. Adequacy of support can be judged during passage of catheters superiorly and toward the LV before attempting to pass the new valve prosthesis.
- The operator must anticipate shortening of the S3 prosthesis toward the LV, and ensure enough of the atrial portion lies within the LA while having the majority of the prosthesis reside in the LV. To enhance stability, balloon postdilatation should be performed to flare the outflow portion of the S3 prosthesis.

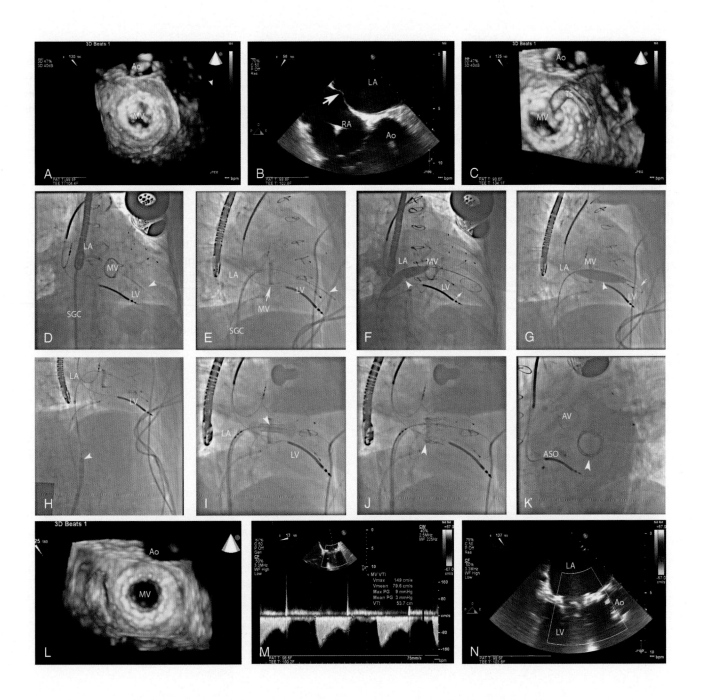

Bioprosthetic Valve Fracture to Facilitate Valve-in-Valve Transcatheter Aortic Valve Replacement

Adnan K. Chhatriwalla, MD

A 77-year-old man with prior surgical aortic valve replacement and coronary bypass surgery presented with severe bioprosthetic aortic stenosis and New York Heart Association class III congestive heart failure (CHF) symptoms. He was felt to be a high-risk surgical candidate, and was recommended for valve-in-valve transcatheter aortic valve replacement (VIV TAVR). A, Aortic root angiography demonstrates a normal sized aortic root and a 23-mm Perimount (Edwards Lifesciences, Irvine, CA) bioprosthetic valve. The patient proceeded to transfemoral VIV TAVR. B and C, The bioprosthetic aortic valve was crossed in retrograde fashion and a 26-mm Corevalve Evolut R (Medtronic Inc., Minneapolis, MN) was successfully positioned and deployed. D, Following VIV TAVR, left heart catheterization demonstrated a mean valve gradient of 27 mm Hg and the effective valve orifice area (EOA) was 0.9 cm^2. Due to suboptimal hemodynamics, bioprosthetic valve fracture (BVF) was performed using a 24-mm True Dilatation balloon (Bard, Tempe, AZ). E, The "waist" of the balloon as it was inflated (arrows). F, The bioprosthetic valve fractured at 16 atm, with full expansion of the balloon noted on fluorscopy (arrows). G, Left heart catheterization following BVF dmeonstrated a mean valve gradient of 9 mm Hg and EOA of 1.7 cm^2. H, The fracture of the bioprosthetic sewing ring can be clearly observed on computed tomography reconstruction (arrow).

Ao, Ascending aorta; LV, left ventricle.

KEY POINTS

- Bioprosthetic valve fracture with a high-pressure balloon can be performed safely in the setting of VIV TAVR in select patients.
- Bioprosthetic valve fracture can improve intraprocedural hemodynamics by decreasing the residual valve gradient and increasing the effective orifice area.

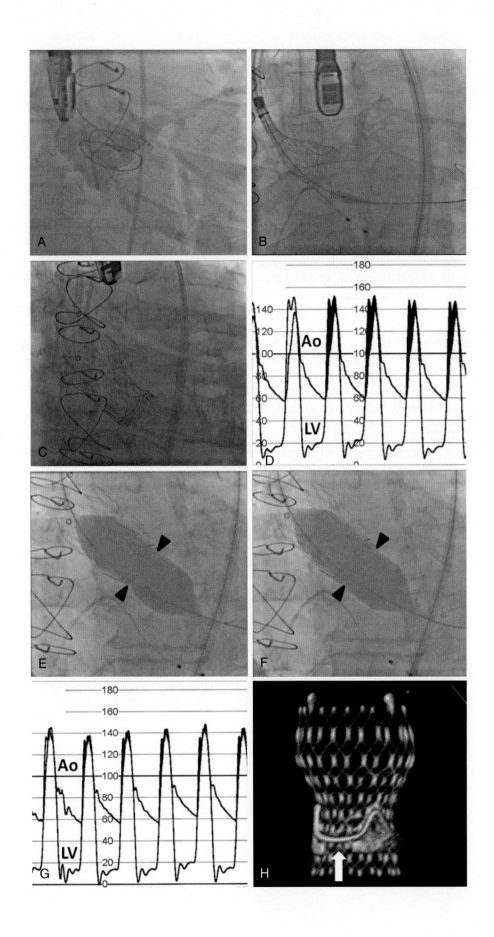

Self-Expanding Prosthesis for Aortic Valve-in-Valve

Paul Sorajja, MD

A 77-year-old woman was referred for transcatheter valve-in-valve therapy of a degenerated prosthesis associated with new symptoms of exertional dyspnea. Seven years ago, she underwent surgery with placement of a 23-mm Edwards Magna prosthesis for severe aortic stenosis. A, Preprocedural imaging with transesophageal echocardiography (TEE) shows the degenerated prosthesis (arrowhead), which was associated with a mean gradient of 74 mm Hg. B, There also was a moderate degree of aortic insufficiency (arrow). C, A 23-mm Evolut R (Medtronic, Dublin, Ireland) was chosen for the procedure (arrowhead) and placed using a retrograde approach from the right femoral artery. D, The prosthesis was implanted at a depth of 2 to 3 mm (arrowhead), thereby maximizing the supra-annular position and effective orifice area. E, On TEE, there was a trivial degree of aortic insufficiency on the short-axis view (arrowhead), and (F) none evident on long-axis imaging. Invasive hemodynamics showed a significant drop in the mean gradient from 82 mm Hg at baseline (G) to only 5 mm Hg after valve implantation (H).

Ao, Ascending aorta; AV, aortic valve; LA, left atrium; LV, left ventricle; RA, right atrium.

KEY POINTS

- The Evolut R prosthesis has a supra-annular design that helps to maximize the effective orifice area and minimize residual gradients, which can be problematic for the treatment of degenerated aortic valve prostheses.
- To maximize the potential hemodynamic benefit with the use of Evolut R for aortic valve-in-valve therapy, the prosthesis should be implanted as high as possible, preferably 3 mm or less.

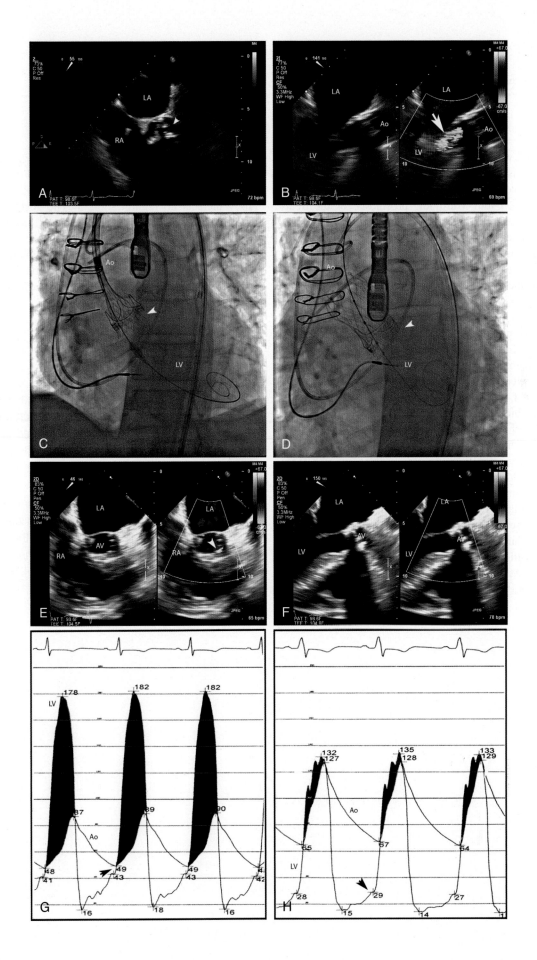

Small Prosthesis Therapy

Paul Sorajja, MD

An 77-year-old woman, with a prior history of aortic valve replacement, was referred for transcatheter therapy of severe symptoms. Six years ago, she underwent cardiac surgery with placement of a 21-mm MitroFlow prosthesis for the treatment of aortic stenosis. Recently, she developed progressive, exertional dyspnea, and an echocardiogram showed a degenerated aortic prosthesis with a mean gradient of 46 mm Hg. A, On cardiac computed tomography (CT), the height from the aortic prosthesis to her right coronary artery was 7.0 mm. B, Imaging with CT also demonstrated the height from the aortic prosthesis to the left coronary artery being 7.2 mm. The Mitroflow prosthesis has externally mounted leaflets, with a height of 14 mm. Thus aortic valve-in-valve therapy carried the potential for coronary obstruction in this patient. C, To help determine this potential, the prosthetic ring is identified on CT imaging (AV) and is traced. D, The tracing of the ring, which represents the maximum diameter after valve-in-valve therapy, is then superimposed at the level of the coronary arteries. The distance of this ring tracing (arrow) to each coronary artery is measured. In this case, the measurements are 3.8 mm for left coronary artery and 3.7 mm for right coronary artery. E, The Evolut R (Ev) prosthesis is partially implanted (arrowhead), and an aortogram is performed to ensure the coronary arteries are patent before final release. F, Because the surgical prosthesis is saddle-shaped, multiple projections are performed to ensure the Evolut R (arrowhead) rests beneath the surgical prosthesis (arrow). In this view, the surgical prosthesis plane is aligned (arrow) with the Evolut R prosthesis beneath it (arrowhead). G, In this view, the Evolut R valve plane (arrowhead) is aligned beneath the surgical prosthesis (arrow). H, Final view shows the complete deployment. I, On transthoracic echocardiography there is no regurgitation. J, The postprocedural gradient across the newly placed Evolut R prosthesis is only 12.6 mm Hg.

Ao, Ascending aorta; AV, surgical aortic valve; Ev, Evolut R; LA, left atirum; LCA, left coronary artery; LV, left ventricle; PA, pulmonary artery; RA, right atrium; RCA, right coronary artery; RV, right ventricle.

KEY POINTS

- The risk of coronary artery obstruction must be considered for patients undergoing aortic valve-in-valve therapy. The risks are increased in surgical valves with externally mounted leaflets (Trifecta, Mitroflow), and those patients with small sinus diameters.
- On cardiac CT, the risk of coronary artery obstruction can be estimated by measuring the distance from the ostia of the arteries to the predicted excursion of the surgical or transcatheter prosthesis. Distances that are ≤3 mm are highest risk of obstruction.

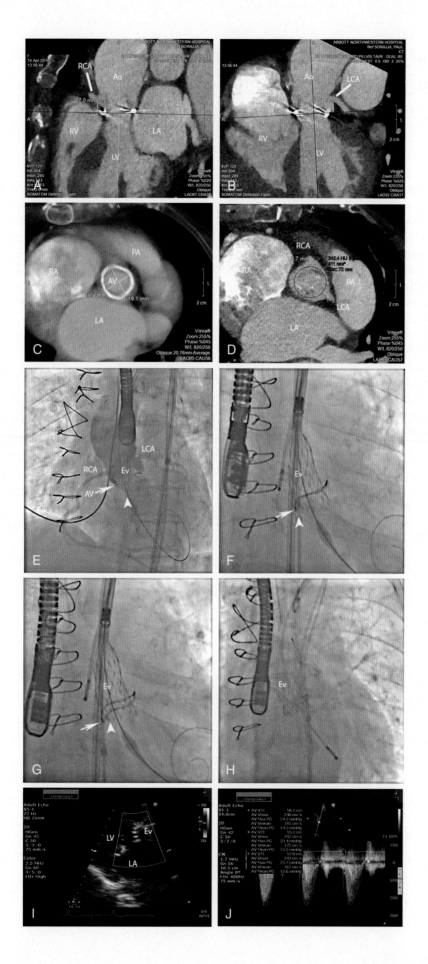

Transcatheter Valve-in-Valve Therapy Utilizing a Melody Valve for Bioprosthetic Tricuspid Valve Failure

Jason H. Anderson, MD, and Allison K. Cabalka, MD

A 71-year-old woman with Ebstein anomaly, who previously underwent bidirectional cavopulmonary anastomosis and tricuspid valve replacement with a 23-mm Medtronic Hancock II bioprosthetic valve (Medtronic, Minneapolis, MN), presented with mixed bioprosthetic valve failure. A femoral venous approach was utilized with placement of a 20-Fr Gore DrySeal Sheath (W.L. Gore & Associates Inc., Newark, DE). A, Intracardiac echocardiography was performed with a 10-Fr AcuNav system (Boston Scientific, San Jose, CA) demonstrating thickened valve leaflets with moderate stenosis (arrows) (mean diastolic inflow gradient = 9 mm Hg). B, There was severe transvalvular regurgitation (arrow) with no paravalvular leak. C and D, A 0.035″ Lunderquist Extra-Stiff Wire Guide (Cook Medical, Bloomington, IN) (arrow) was placed in the distal right pulmonary artery with the valve profiled in the (C) right anterior oblique (RAO) and (D) left anterior oblique (LAO) imaging planes. E, Balloon sizing of the bioprosthetic valve with a 22-mm Z-med II balloon (B. Braun Medical Inc., Bethlehem, PA) demonstrated a 20-mm minimum internal diameter (arrow). F–H, A 22-mm Melody transcatheter heart valve (F, arrow) (Medtronic, Minneapolis, MN) was delivered on a 22-mm Ensemble delivery system (G, arrow) (Medtronic) within the existing bioprosthesis in the tricuspid valve position (H, arrow). I, Postimplantation intracardiac echocardiography demonstrated thin leaflets with normal mobility and coaptation (arrows). J, Trivial central regurgitation was present (arrow) with no stenosis or paravalvular leak. The patient had relief of right-sided heart failure symptoms, obviating the need for open surgery.

RA, Right atrium; RV, right ventricle.

KEY POINTS

- In select cases of tricuspid bioprosthetic valve failure, transcatheter valve-in-valve therapy is a viable alternative to surgical valve replacement.
- The Melody valve is available in 18- to 22-mm sizes and is more commonly selected for congenital cases and bioprosthetic valves with a smaller internal diameter (≤24 mm).

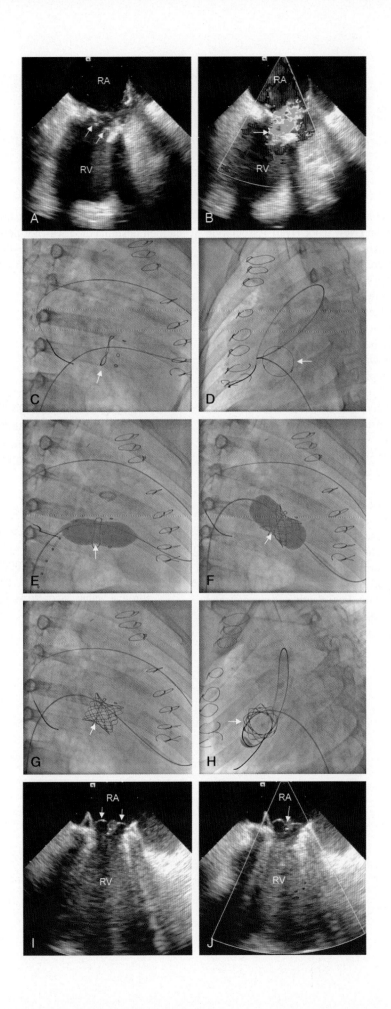

Valve-in-Valve Transcatheter Aortic Valve Replacement With a Repositionable, Self-Expanding Valve

Ankur Kalra, MD, Neal S. Kleiman, MD, Colin M. Barker, MD, and Michael J. Reardon, MD

An 89-year-old woman presented for evaluation of progressive dyspnea on exertion (New York Heart Association Class III). Eighteen years ago, she underwent surgical aortic valve replacement for severe aortic stenosis with a 21-mm Carpentier-Edwards prosthesis. A 2-dimensional echocardiogram demonstrated severe thickening and calcification of the bioprosthetic aortic valve leaflets. The peak aortic valve velocity was 4.5 m/s with a mean gradient of 53 mm Hg, a calculated valve area of 0.5 cm^2, and a Doppler velocity index of <0.25. The patient was scheduled for a transfemoral, transcatheter aortic valve replacement with a repositionable, self-expanding CoreValve Evolut R 26-mm valve (Medtronic, Inc., Minneapolis, MN). Valve sizing was determined based on the true internal dimension of the Carpentier-Edwards bioprosthetic valve and the sinus of Valsalva diameter (all sinuses measured >27 mm) (A and B). The prosthetic valve was crossed with an amplatz left-2 catheter, and a 0.035″, 150-cm straight-tip crossing wire, followed by recording of the left ventricular and aortic pressures (peak-to-peak gradient, 40 mm Hg; C and D). Balloon aortic valvuloplasty was not performed prior to transcatheter valve-in-valve deployment. The transcatheter Evolut R was intentionally deployed high in relation to the bioprosthetic valve annulus to minimize residual gradients and maximize the effective orifice area (target depth = 0 to 2 mm; final depth = 2 mm) (E and F). The post-deployment peak-to-peak left ventricle to aorta gradient was 0 mm Hg (C and D), with a Doppler velocity index of 0.79. There was no paravalvular regurgitation, and balloon postdilatation was not performed.

Ao, Aortic; CE, Carpentier-Edwards; LV, left ventricular; SoV, sinus of Valsalva; TAVR, transcatheter aortic valve replacement.

KEY POINTS

- Targeting a relatively high implant depth for valve-in-valve aortic procedures helps to minimize residual gradients from transcatheter therapy, particularly for the treatment of small surgical bioprostheses.
- When small prostheses are present, the aortic diameters should be adequately large to allow full expansion of the outflow segment of the transcatheter prosthesis.
- Postdilation, following transcatheter valve-in-valve replacement, if required, should be based on the surgical valve size to facilitate stretching of the surgical valve ring.

ANNULUS   SOV DIAMETER

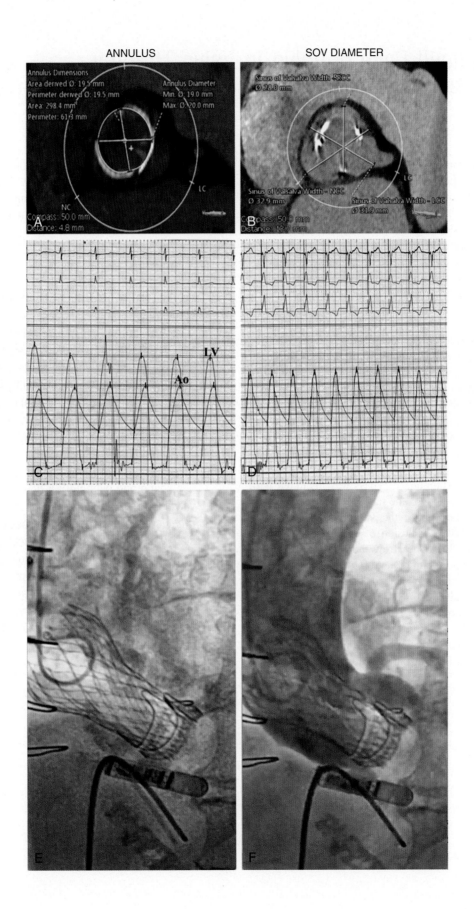

A Very Difficult Case of Valve-in-Valve Therapy

Joy S. Shome, MBBS, MRCP, Rizwan Attia, PhD, MRCS, and Vinayak N. Bapat, MCh, FRCS(CTh)

A, A 76-year-old-woman presented with exertional angina and decompensated heart failure due to a failing, 11-year-old, 21-mm Mitraflow aortic valve bioprosthesis (Sorin Group, London, United Kingdom), which originally had been implanted for degenerative aortic stenosis. B, Transthoracic echocardiography confirmed severe stenosis and regurgitation due to bioprosthesis degeneration. Coronary angiography showed only mild coronary artery atheroma. She was considered for valve-in-valve transcatheter aortic valve replacement (VIV TAVR) due to high surgical risk. She underwent transfemoral VIV TAVR using an Edwards Sapien 20 mm XT prosthesis (Edwards Lifesciences, Irvine, CA). C, After deployment, there was catastrophic hemodynamic collapse, and aortography revealed hypoperfused coronary arteries with an occluded right coronary artery (RCA) and partially occluded left main stem (LMS). D, Emergency percutaneous coronary intervention to the RCA ostium was performed, but (E) the LMS could not be wired and there was subsequent cardiac arrest. With cardiopulmonary resuscitation ongoing, the patient was transferred to the operating theater and cardiopulmonary bypass was instituted with improvement in her hemodynamic status. F, Redo-sternotomy was performed. Inspection of the valve-in-valve complex after aortotomy revealed occlusion of the coronary arteries by the Mitraflow leaflets. The arrow indicates the left main stem ostium at the sino-tubular junction, which was occluded by the leaflets of Mitraflow valve (M) after the implantation of the Sapien XT valve (S). G, The Sapien and Mitraflow valves were both explanted. After explanting the Sapien XT, the leaflet of the Mitraflow valve (M) was retracted to demonstrate the left main ostium (black arrow), confirming obstruction of blood flow in this location. After aortic root enlargement, a 19-mm Magna Ease aortic valve bioprosthesis (Edwards Lifesciences, Irvine, CA) was implanted. The postoperative course was uneventful, and the patient made a complete recovery with improvement in symptoms.

KEY POINTS

- Valve-in-valve procedure always carries a risk of coronary obstruction. Patients with a small aortic root and narrow sinuses of Valsalva are particularly susceptible. The surgical valve design is also important, with valves whose leaflets are outside the stent frame having significantly higher risk.
- Bioprosthetic valve anatomy and the associated risk of coronary obstruction can be assessed with a gated computed tomography scan or careful assessment of the fluoroscopic characteristics of the aortic root and sino-tubular junction (i.e., relative shape and diameter). If doubt persists, balloon valvuloplasty with simultaneous aortic root angiography can be performed to assess coronary perfusion with expansion of the surgical prosthesis.
- If the risk of coronary obstruction is high, protection by prewiring, with or without a stent, and use of standby circulatory support are helpful. Prompt institution of cardiopulmonary bypass can give the operator time to treat the complication with either stenting or redo-surgery.

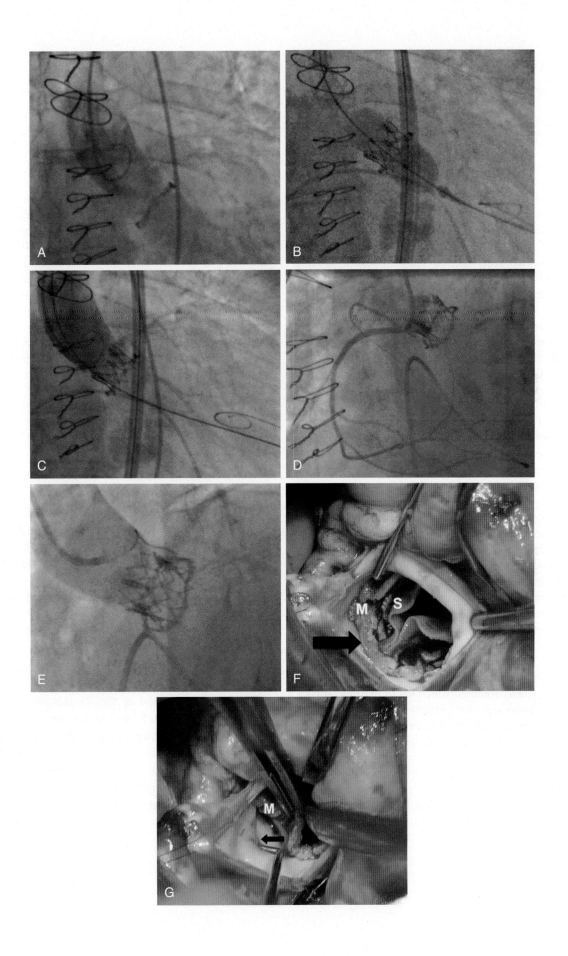

Antegrade Balloon-Expandable Valve for Tricuspid Valve-in-Valve Therapy

Paul Sorajja, MD

A 54-year-old woman with multiple, severe comorbidities presented for treatment of a degenerated tricuspid valve prosthesis. Six years ago, she underwent tricuspid surgery with placement of a 31-mm Epic prosthesis (St. Jude Medical, Fridley, MN). Two years ago, the patient began to develop symptoms of right heart failure that were refractory to medical therapy. A, A transthoracic echocardiogram showed a well-seated tricuspid prosthesis (arrow) and a mean gradient of 10.2 mm Hg on Doppler imaging. B, 3-dimensional (3-D) echocardiogram with an en face view from the right atrium (RA) demonstrates the tricuspid prosthesis with stenosis (TV). C, Using an approach from the right femoral vein, a balloon wedge (BW) catheter is advanced through the tricuspid prosthesis (arrowheads) to the right pulmonary artery. This location was chosen for the wire as her right ventricle (RV) was small, and there was concern there would not be enough stiffness with placement in the RV. For rapid ventricular pacing, a multipurpose (MP) catheter is placed into the left ventricle, followed by placement of a 2 Fr active fixation, temporary pacemaker lead (arrow). D, A 260-cm, Super Stiff wire is placed through the balloon wedge catheter into the pulmonary vascular bed (arrow). E, A 29-mm Sapien S3 prosthesis (S; Edwards Lifesciences, Irvine, CA) is positioned with the deployment marker on the surgical prosthesis ring (arrowheads), anticipating that shortening of the prosthesis will occur in the ventricular direction. Assembly onto the deployment balloon is performed with the delivery catheter in the inferior vena cava. At this point, the prosthesis has a superior orientation and cannot be corrected with various maneuvers, including full flexion, retraction toward the RA (due to the prosthesis being stuck on the surgical valve), catheter rotation (which led to twisting, arrow), or forward advancement (due to concern that atrial positioning would be lost). F, The Stiff Wire (arrowheads) is then pushed to bring the catheter as inferior as possible (arrow). The delivery catheter is then retracted past the marker (M) for more orientation from the wire. G, Further tension is applied to the wire (arrowheads) and the S3 prosthesis is deployed with rapid ventricular pacing. Care is taken to ensure that a portion of the atrial component of the S3 prosthesis remains on the atrial side of the surgical valve. H, Following removal of the delivery catheter and wire, the S3 prosthesis (arrows) self-orients in the surgical prosthesis. I, Transesophageal echocardiography demonstrates trivial regurgitation (arrowhead). J, 3-D echocardiography shows deployed S3 prosthesis with relief of the stenosis. The final gradient across the tricuspid prosthesis is 4 mm Hg. The right femoral vein is closed with two previously placed Proglide sutures for complete hemostasis.

BW, Balloon wedge; MP, multipurpose catheter; RA, right atrium; RV, right ventricle; RVOT, right ventricular outflow tract; S, S3 prosthesis.

KEY POINTS

- For patients requiring tricuspid valve-in-valve therapy, the RV may be small in size. Placement of the guidewire in the pulmonary artery may be required to ensure the stiff segment is across the prosthesis for support. Positioning in the right lung field provides a large, single guidewire loop for use during the procedure.
- Using the pulmonary artery for guidewire placement can lead to a superior orientation of the prosthesis during positioning. This superior orientation can be overcome with tension applied to the guidewire, as well as the self-orienting nature of the prosthesis once it is deployed.
- The inflow portion of the S3 prosthesis shortens during deployment, and care must be undertaken to ensure the atrial portion of the S3 prosthesis is secure on the atrial side of the surgical prosthesis. Balloon post-dilatation may be required to flare the outflow portion of the prosthesis, thereby promoting a cork-like effect for stability.

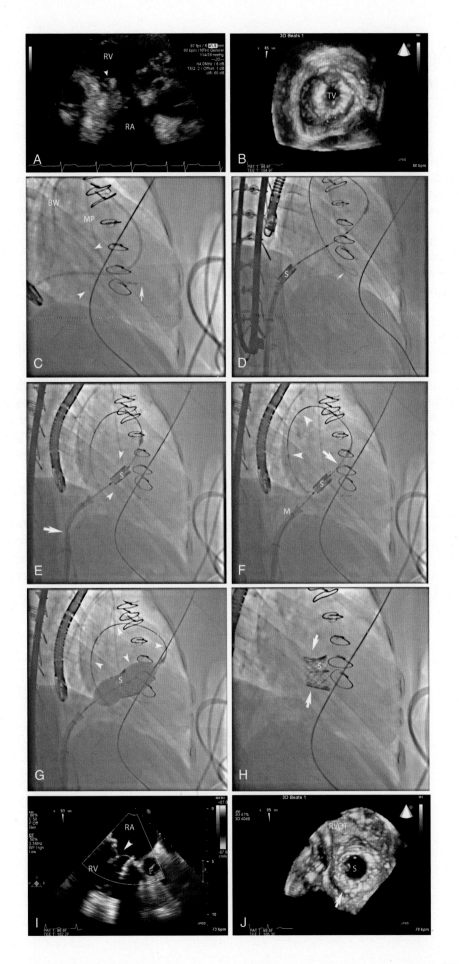

Complex Tricuspid Valve-in-Valve Therapy

Gilbert H. L. Tang, MD, MSc, MBA, Hasan Ahmad, MD, and Martin Cohen, MD

A 49-year-old frail woman presented with severe heart failure, liver congestion, and ascites. In 1993, she underwent cardiac surgery with placement of bioprostheses in the aortic, mitral, and tricuspid positions. In 2006, she had reoperative mechanical aortic and mitral valve replacements. A, Her current echocardiogram demonstrated prosthetic tricuspid stenosis with a mean gradient of 21 mm Hg. The patient was considered prohibitive surgical risk, and further evaluation for tricuspid valve-in-valve (T-VIV) therapy was undertaken. The size of the tricuspid bioprosthesis was unknown, but a 31-mm Carpentier-Edwards porcine bioprosthesis was suspected based on (B) computed tomography and (C) fluoroscopy with size calculations derived from both mechanical valves. A 29-mm Edwards Sapien XT valve (Edwards Lifesciences, Irvine, CA) was planned for T-VIV. Given the uncertainty about the size of the tricuspid bioprosthesis, balloon valvuloplasty with the 29-mm Novaflex+ delivery catheter was used for sizing, to assess balloon movement and stability, and as a "dry run" for valve positioning and deployment. D, An Amplatz Super Stiff wire was positioned at the distal right pulmonary artery for support. Balloon valvuloplasty was performed without rapid ventricular pacing and balloon "waisting" could be seen, indicating that a 29-mm Sapien XT valve would be appropriate for T-VIV implantation. The Sapien XT valve, mounted in its usual aortic orientation, was advanced to the tricuspid bioprosthesis with the Edwards logo on the delivery catheter facing down. E, During the deployment, real-time adjustment of the Novaflex+ delivery flex-cath wheel knob optimized coaxiality of the transcatheter valve relative to the bioprosthesis, without incurring excessive tension in the system. F, Valve implantation was successful and the patient was discharged home uneventfully. An echocardiogram at 18-month follow-up showed no central or paravalvular regurgitation, and the mean gradient was 2 mm Hg.

KEY POINTS

- Balloon valvuloplasty for sizing can be performed when there is uncertainty regarding appropriate prosthesis size.
- Appropriate flexion and positioning during T-VIV therapy with the Edwards prosthesis is facilitated with a stiff wire in the right pulmonary artery, inverting the delivery sheath (logo facing down), and applying and relieving tension via the flex cath wheel.
- Patients with prosthetic tricuspid valve failure carry dismal prognosis and are extremely high to prohibitive risk for reoperative surgery.
- Transcatheter tricuspid valve-in-valve replacement with balloon-expandable valve offers a minimally invasive and effective option for these patients.

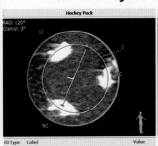

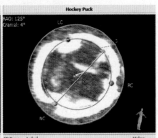

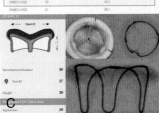

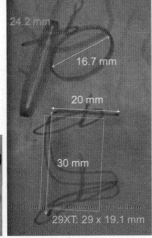

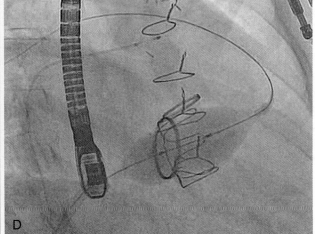

Valve Deployment with Real-Time Flex-cath Wheel Adjustment

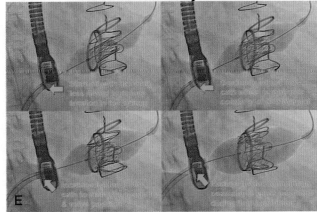

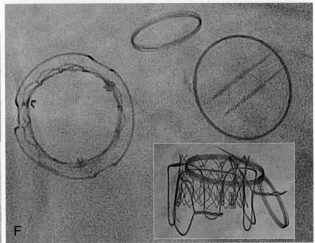

Fusion Imaging for Percutaneous Transapical Access

Tilak K. R. Pasala, MD, Vladimir Jelnin, MD, and Carlos E. Ruiz, MD

Percutaneous transapical access allows access to the left ventricle, mitral valve, and aortic valve for a variety of structural heart disease procedures without the need for a surgical cut down. Fluoroscopy alone does not provide characterization of soft tissues, and is limited by 2-dimensional projection of 3-dimensional (3-D) anatomy. By integrating computed tomography angiography (CTA) and fluoroscopy, (CTA-Fluoroscopy fusion), a controlled transapical access with high success and safety can be performed. Careful procedural planning is paramount and can be done by specialized software (Heart Navigator, Philips Healthcare, Inc.). Initially, various cardiac structures are identified on the standard anatomical planes (axial, sagittal, and coronal), and designated color mesh is applied automatically (A). Then a 3-D model is created (B), and the intended target is marked. Importantly, a "safe path" from the access site on the skin to the target is built by avoiding left anterior descending artery and lungs (B–C). The left ventricular apex, which is thin-walled should be avoided. The pre-processed CTA images are then co-registered to scale and orientation with live fluoroscopy. The C-arm angle is rotated to a point, where the safe path is seen as a circle (D, black arrow). A long micropuncture needle is steered toward the target through the circle. The depth of the needle can be checked by rotating the C-arm (E). After the procedure, the left ventricular puncture site is closed with an Amplatzer Vascular Type II plug (St. Jude Medical, St. Paul, MN) (E).

KEY POINTS

- Percutaneous transapical access can be performed effectively and safely with careful, detailed preprocedural planning with advanced imaging.
- Device closure of the percutaneous left ventricular access is recommended.

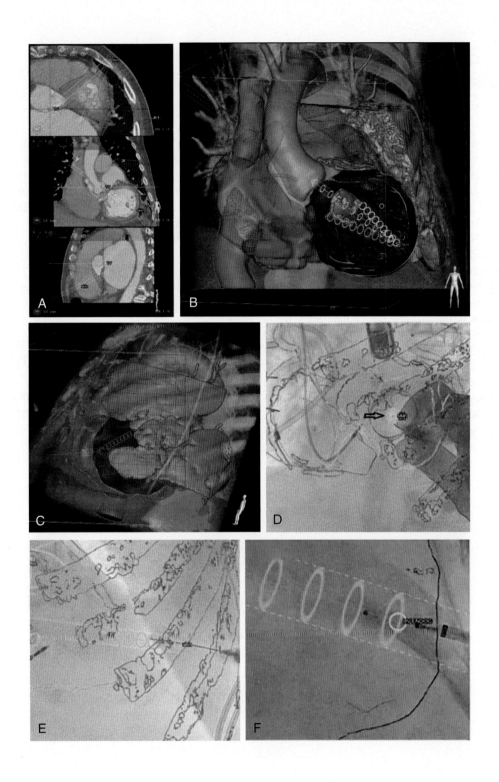

Fusion Imaging for Mitral Valve-in-Valve Replacement

Tilak K. R. Pasala, MD, Vladimir Jelnin, MD, and Carlos E. Ruiz, MD, PhD

An 85-year-old woman with a prior history of mitral valve (MV) replacement with a 25-mm Edwards Perimount prosthesis (Edwards Lifesciences, Irvine, CA) presented with shortness of breath on exertion. Echocardiography and computed tomography angiography (CTA) showed abnormal leaflet function of mitral bioprosthesis, and severe mitral regurgitation. A, Using specialized software, a segmented 3-dimensional model of the heart was built for preprocedural planning and intraprocedural guidance (Fusion imaging). B, First, transapical access was obtained using a micropuncture needle, and a 6-Fr, 23-cm radial sheath (Cook Medical, Bloomington, IN) was placed into the cardiac apex using CTA-Fluoroscopy fusion. An Edwards sheath was placed in the right atrium. Transseptal access was obtained in standard fashion, and a long stiff Glidewire (Terumo, Somerset, NJ) was placed in the left atrium. Then, a JR4 guide and 18 × 30-mm Ensnare (Merit Medical Systems Inc., South Jordan, UT) was advanced through the transapical sheath. C, The glidewire was snared and externalized through the MV prosthesis, creating an arterial-venous rail (white arrows). D,

After an atrial septostomy, a 26-mm Sapien XT valve and delivery system (Edwards Lifesciences, Irvine, CA) was advanced over the antegrade, over the rail, across the MV, under fusion imaging. The yellow line marked the deployment angle. E, The Sapien valve was deployed (arrow) and (F) final position was checked (arrow).

MV, Mitral valve; RA, right atrium.

KEY POINTS

- Fusion imaging can be useful for safe, transapical access to create an arteriovenous rail for support in mitral valve-in-valve therapies.
- Fusion imaging provides orientation of the cardiac structures on fluoroscopy to facilitate access, catheter manipulation, and placement of devices.

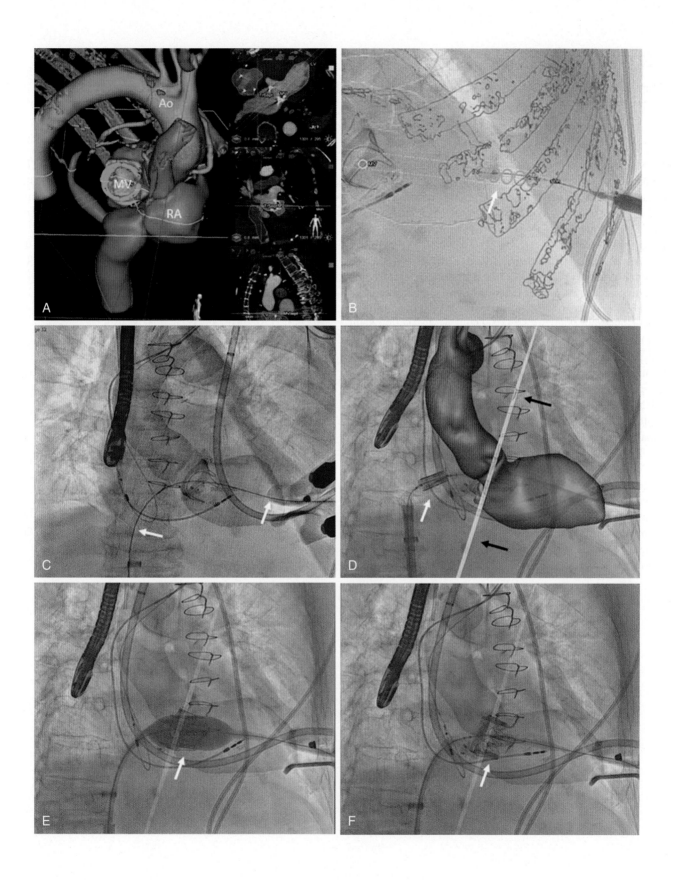

Challenging Case of Surgical Mitral Ring Therapy

Brandon M. Jones, MD, Amar Krishnaswamy, MD, and Samir R. Kapadia, MD

A 58-year-old man presented with severe, progressive heart failure in the setting of prior radiation therapy for Hodgkin's disease, fibrosing pleuritis with recurrent pleural effusions, and prior coronary artery bypass surgery and mitral valve (MV) repair with a #28 Classic Edwards Ring (Edwards Lifescience, Irvine, CA). He was found to have severe mitral stenosis with a mean gradient of 12 mm Hg at rest, and his symptoms were refractory to medical therapy. Due to his severe comorbidity, he was determined not to be a candidate for repeat open heart surgery. The patient was brought to the hybrid operating room, where transseptal access was obtained and balloon septostomy performed. A balloon-tipped catheter was passed across the mitral orifice, and a stiff wire advanced through the left ventricle, across the aortic valve, and into the descending aorta. A and B, A 29-mm Edwards Sapien XT valve (arrow; Edwards Lifesciences, Irvine, CA) was deployed inside the prior mitral ring, but there was severe, dynamic left ventricular outflow tract (LVOT) obstruction. C and D, Additional access was obtained in the femoral artery and balloon dilation of the LVOT was performed (arrows), without improvement in the obstruction. E and F, Alcohol septal ablation was then performed on the first septal perforator branch of the left anterior descending coronary artery (arrows), resulting in the elimination of the LVOT gradient. Imaging with transesophageal echocardiography (G) before and (H) after septal ablation demonstrated LVOT obstruction at baseline that improved with the procedure (arrows). There was no further septal contact between the native MV leaflets and the ventricular septum. Invasive hemodynamic evaluations (I) before and (J) after the septal ablation confirmed relief of the LVOT obstruction.

Ao, Ascending aorta; G, left coronary guide catheter; LA, left atrium; LV, left ventricle; S, Sapien XT valve; TPM, temporary pacemaker; VS, ventricular septum.

KEY POINTS

- When performing transcatheter mitral valve-in-valve or valve-in-ring procedures, one must be aware of the potential for creating life-threatening LVOT obstruction.
- Risk factors for LVOT obstruction with transcatheter mitral valve therapy are small left ventricular cavity, septal hypertrophy, large size of mitral prosthesis, and acute angle of the aorta-mitral curtain.
- Treatment options for LVOT obstruction include balloon dilation of the LVOT and alcohol septal ablation in appropriate cases.

200 PROSTHETIC VALVE

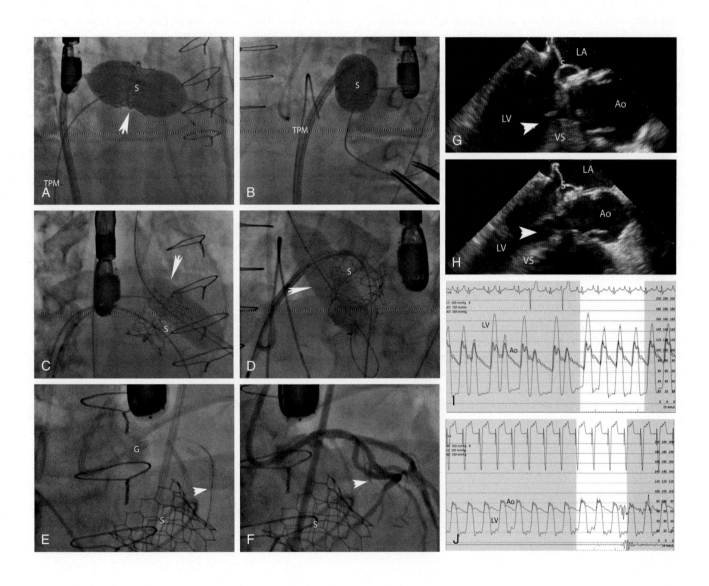

Left Ventricular Outflow Tract Obstruction and Severe Reversible Ventricular Dysfunction After Valve-in-Ring Mitral Replacement

Mark V. Sherrid, Muhamed Saric, MD, PhD, and Mathew R. Williams, MD

An 88-year-old woman developed heart failure ten years after prior mitral valvuloplasty and a placement of a mitral annuloplasty ring. On transesophageal echocardiography (TEE), severe mitral regurgitation (MR) with thickening of the mitral leaflets was evident. After consideration of the options, she underwent transcatheter, valve-in-ring (VIR) mitral replacement with a Sapien 3 valve (Edwards Lifesciences, Irvine, CA).

A–C, Following placement of the Sapien prosthesis, there was hemodynamic instability. TEE showed a well-seated prosthesis and ring, with marked reduction in MR and no paravalvular regurgitation. However, there was systolic anterior motion (SAM) of the retained residual anterior mitral leaflet, with severe left ventricular outflow tract (LVOT) obstruction (arrow, A, transgastric, short-axis TEE in diastole; arrow, B, transgastric, short-axis TEE in systole; C, 3-chamber TEE view in systole; red arrows show SAM; yellow arrows indicate mitral prosthesis). The LVOT gradient was 174 mm Hg on short-axis, transgastric TEE imaging.

Intravenous fluids and beta-blockers were administered that incompletely reduced the LVOT gradient. D and E, The next day, new left ventricular dilatation and severe systolic dysfunction was noted on transthoracic echocardiography (4-chamber views in diastole and systole, respectively).

After 3 weeks, there was persistent left ventricular dysfunction, ventricular and atrial arrhythmias, and severe exercise intolerance. F, On transthoracic echocardiography, there was SAM with mitral-septal contact and mid-systolic aortic valve closure (red arrows; mitral prosthesis, yellow arrows).

She then underwent AV nodal ablation and insertion of a biventricular pacemaker to regularize her RR intervals. A VV interval of 50 msec from left ventricle to right ventricle was most effective in lowering the LVOT gradient. H, Her LVOT gradient resolved and the left ventricular ejection fraction normalized (65%), in conjunction with functional status improvement to minimal residual symptoms.

Ao, Ascending aorta.

KEY POINTS

- LVOT obstruction may complicate percutaneous VIR mitral valve replacement due to the anterior displacement of the residual native mitral anterior leaflet.
- Hemodynamic effects of LVOT obstruction can result in severe left ventricular systolic dysfunction.
- Ventricular pacing may induce ventricular dyssynchrony and improve LVOT obstruction, and can be effective for refractory cases.
- Promotion of AV synchrony and regularization of the RR intervals also may be effective therapies.

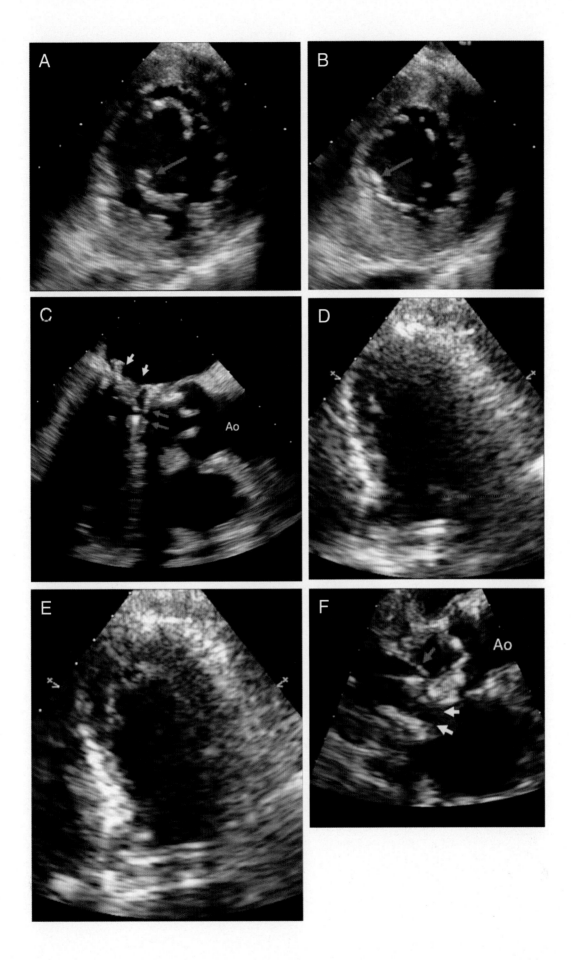

Cardiomyopathy

Reversed Pulsus Paradoxus

Paul Sorajja, MD

Reversed pulsus paradoxus occurs in patients with obstructive hypertrophic cardiomyopathy (HCM) and needs to be distinguished from cardiac tamponade. These are simultaneous assessments of ascending aortic and left ventricular pressures in a patient with obstructive HCM. Note the dynamic nature of the left ventricular outflow tract (LVOT) gradient even during quiet respiration. During expiration, positive thoracic pressure leads to a decrease in afterload, followed by increases in the LVOT gradient. Conversely, inspiration augments afterload, and thereby decreases LVOT obstruction, followed by a *rise* in the aortic pulse pressure. These changes are not mediated by preload alterations. In cardiac tamponade, there is pulsus paradoxus, which is indicated by an inspiratory decrease in the aortic pulse pressure. The expiratory and inspiratory phases of respiration in these patients are indicated by the changes in ventricular diastolic pressure or atrial pressures.

Ao, Ascending aorta; LV, left ventricle.

KEY POINTS

- Reversed pulsus paradoxus occurs in obstructive HCM due to changes in ventricular afterload during respiration.
- Knowing the onset of expiration and inspiration, as indicated by the ventricular diastolic filling pressures, is the key to differentiating pulsus paradoxus due to cardiac tamponade from reverse pulsus paradoxus due to obstructive hypertrophic cardiomyopathy.

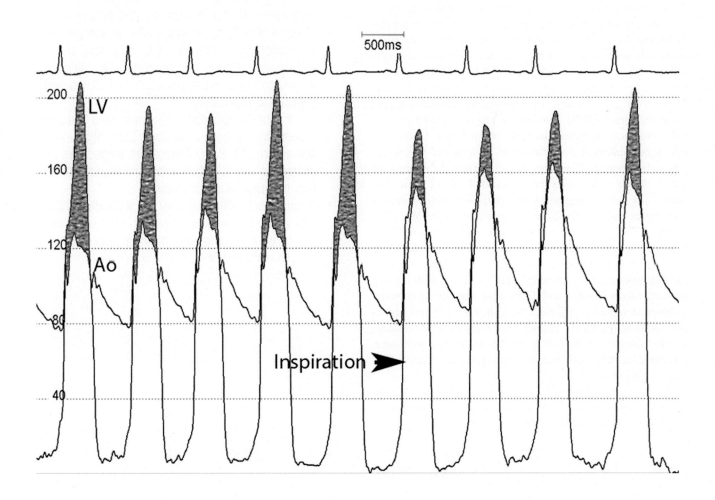

Percutaneous Mitral Valve Repair in Hypertrophic Cardiomyopathy

Paul Sorajja, MD

A 77-year-old woman was referred for treatment of severe, drug-refractory symptoms due to obstructive hypertrophic cardiomyopathy (HCM). She was initially referred for alcohol septal ablation, and elected to undergo percutaneous mitral valve (MV) plication with MitraClip (Abbott Vascular, Santa Clara, CA) in a novel approach to treat these patients. A, Baseline transthoracic echocardiogram with a parasternal long-axis view showing severe myocardial hypertrophy involving the ventricular septum (VS). B, Systolic image from TTE with an apical long-axis view demonstrating systolic anterior motion (SAM) of the MV (arrowhead) and left ventricular outflow tract (LVOT) obstruction. C, The peak LVOT gradient was 146 mm Hg. D, Transesophageal echocardiogram (TEE) showing severe mitral regurgitation (MR) that was secondary to SAM (arrowhead). E, Using a transseptal approach, a single MitraClip is placed (arrow). F, Three-dimensional TEE from the left atrium (i.e., surgeon's view) showing the tissue bridge created by the MitraClip across the A2-P2 segments. G, TEE with color-compare imaging at end-systole shows the position of the MitraClip on the A2-P2 segments (arrowheads), normal laminar flow through the LVOT, and the absence of any residual SAM. H, Color-flow Doppler imaging with TEE in a commissural view demonstrates complete elimination of MR with the clip in place (arrowhead). I and J, Invasive hemodynamic study at baseline and after clip placement shows significant reductions in both the LVOT gradient and the left atrial pressure. Cardiac output, as measured by thermodilution technique, increased acutely with percutaneous plication from 3.3 L/min to 5.0 L/min.

Ao, Ascending aorta; CO, cardiac output; LA, left atrium; LAP, left atrial pressure; LV, left ventricle; RV, right ventricle; VS, ventricular septum.

KEY POINTS

- Percutaneous plication of the MV leaflets can be used to treat dynamic LVOT obstruction in patients with drug-refractory symptoms due to HCM. The technique is similar to methods used for treatment of patients with degenerative MR. In comparison to alcohol septal ablation, this approach, which is largely reversible and repositionable, has the advantages of avoiding myocardial infarction and pacemaker dependency.
- When considering suitable anatomy, ideal features include the presence of dynamic LVOT obstruction and severe MR. Both of these pathologies can be addressed with plication and their alleviation can lead to symptom improvement.
- Patients with MR secondary to obstructive HCM may have relatively smaller left atria, and this should be a consideration during manipulation of the clip delivery system during the procedure.

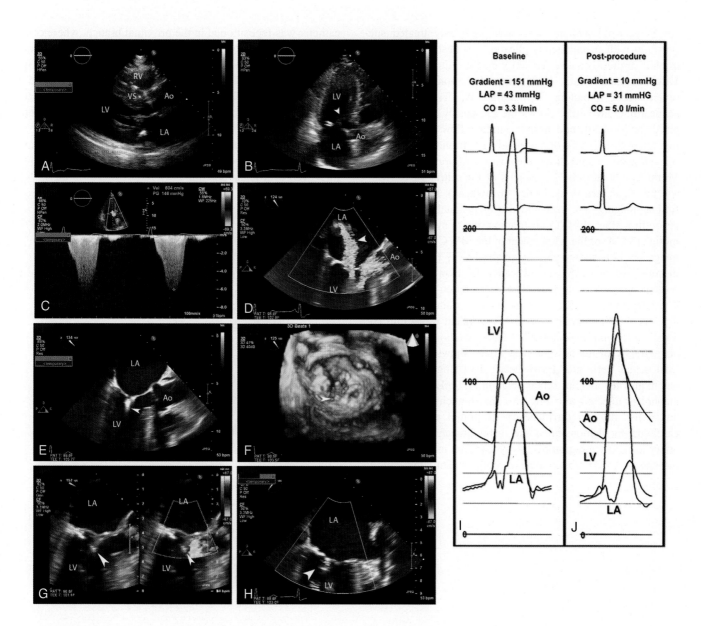

Recurrent Obstruction After Percutaneous Plication in Hypertrophic Cardiomyopathy

Paul Sorajja, MD

An 82-year-old woman, who was previously treated successfully with percutaneous plication for obstructive hypertrophic cardiomyopathy (HCM) with the MitraClip (Abbott Vascular, Santa Clara, CA), returned 9 months later with severe, drug-refractory symptoms. A, Transesophageal echocardiogram (TEE) shows the previously placed clip in place (arrowhead), and normal laminar flow near its position (arrow). B, Three-dimensional TEE from the left atrium (i.e., surgeon's view) shows the position of previously placed MitraClip on the A2-P2 segments of the mitral valve (MV) and the associated tissue bridge (arrowhead). However, with further imaging, she had evidence of residual left ventricular outflow tract (LVOT) obstruction due to systolic anterior motion (SAM) of the A1 segment of the MV. C, End-diastolic image on TEE shows patency of the LVOT (arrow) during diastole and no SAM (arrowheads). D, However, SAM is present during systole with flow acceleration (arrowheads). The lateral mitral orifice was too small for additional percutaneous plication, and her mean MV gradient was 4 mm Hg. She therefore underwent alcohol septal ablation. E, Coronary angiography of the left coronary artery shows a large proximal septal perforator (arrowhead). F, Using conventional techniques for alcohol septal ablation, 1.7 mL of desiccated alcohol is injected into this proximal branch of this septal artery for ablation (arrowhead). G, Initial contrast echocardiography demonstrated the distal branch of the septal artery to supply a region of the myocardium too remote from the site of LVOT obstruction (arrow). H, Thus the balloon catheter was repositioned in the proximal branch, where contrast injection demonstrated an appropriate location for the ablation. I, At baseline, the LVOT gradient was 140 mm Hg with a mean left atrial pressure of 32 mm Hg. J, Following alcohol septal ablation, the LVOT gradient decreased to 10 mm Hg, in association with a reduction of the mean left atrial pressure to 22 mm Hg.

Ao, Ascending aorta; LA, left atrium; LAP, left atrial pressure; LV, left ventricle; LVOT, left ventricular outflow tract; VS, ventricular septum.

KEY POINTS

- While percutaneous plication of the MV with Mitra-Clip can be successful in patients with obstructive HCM, residual SAM may occur and lead to significant LVOT obstruction. These patients can be challenging to treat due to the relatively small size of the mitral orifice, which may not permit placement of more than one clip.
- In selected cases, alcohol septal ablation can be performed to treat residual LVOT obstruction that becomes evident after percutaneous plication with MitraClip.

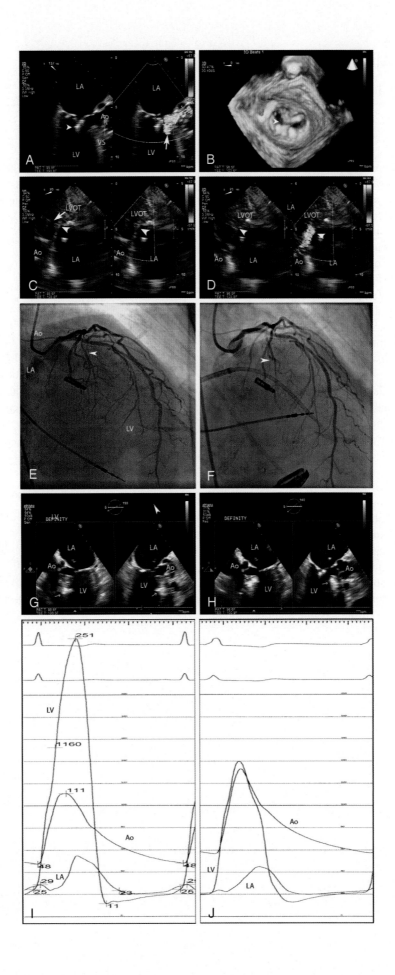

Complicated Alcohol Septal Ablation

Ryan K. Kaple, MD, and Srihari S. Naidu, MD

A 68-year-old man with hypertrophic obstructive cardiomyopathy presented with New York Heart Association class II heart failure symptoms and recurrent pre-syncope. His past medical history included recent coronary artery bypass surgery with concomitant mitral valve (MV) ring annuloplasty. There was ventricular septal hypertrophy with an end-diastolic wall thickness of 2.6 cm. A and B, The left ventricular outflow tract (LVOT) gradient was only 10 mm Hg at rest, but increased to 180 mm Hg with provocation and systolic anterior motion of the anterior MV leaflet. C and D, Coronary angiography demonstrated significant atherosclerosis in the proximal left anterior descending (LAD) artery before the take-off of the first major septal perforator, which had been bypassed by the left internal mammary artery. The first septal perforator also had significant disease at the ostium. Alcohol septal ablation was undertaken. E and F, Attempts to pass a balloon into the septal artery were not initially successful due to the two tandem lesions; thus, balloon angioplasty was performed in the proximal LAD and the ostial septal perforator using a 2.5- × 6.0-mm Sprinter balloon (Medtronic Inc., Mounds View, MN). G–I, Subsequently, the wire was successfully exchanged for an over-the-wire 2.0- × 10-mm Flextome cutting balloon (Boston Scientific, Maple Grove, MN). Myocardial contrast was injected through the balloon lumen to confirm that the branch supplied the hypertrophied segment on echocardiography. A total of 3.0 cc of ethanol was then injected, abolishing the resting and provocable gradients. Postprocedure transthoracic echocardiography demonstrated resolution of the systolic anterior motion (SAM), as well as akinesis of the basal septum. Follow-up echocardiography at two months and two years post-ablation showed no residual LVOT gradient nor SAM, with a septal thickness of only 1.6 cm at two years (J).

KEY POINTS

- Severe mitral regurgitation (MR), with or without coronary artery disease (CAD), may be due to obstructive hypertrophic cardiomyopathy. In operative candidates, a careful assessment of MR in the setting of asymmetric septal hypertrophy is warranted to determine the need for concomitant mitral surgery.
- Surgical mitral annuloplasty, due to changes in position of the valve leaflets, may produce or exacerbate LVOT obstruction.
- Balloon angioplasty may be required to gain access to septal perforators in the setting of severe native CAD.
- Cutting balloons may be utilized in septal perforators measuring ≥2.0 mm in diameter, and may aid in stabilization of both the balloon and guide without the need for extra-support catheters.

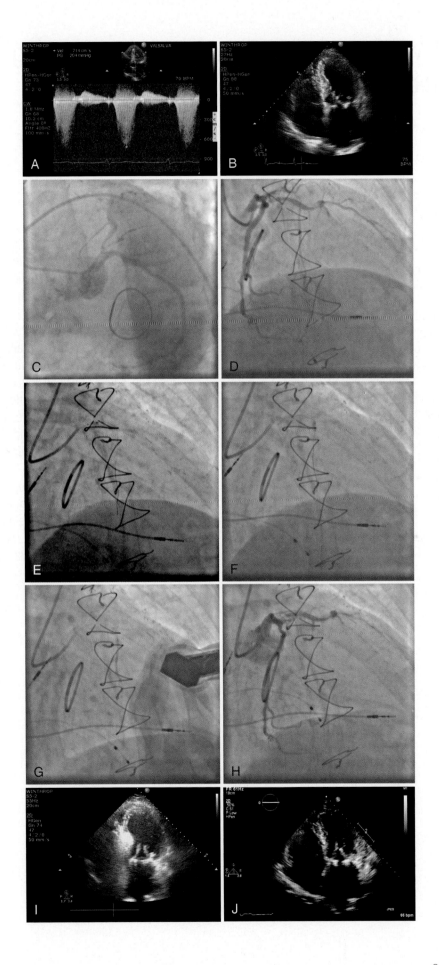

Untoward Myocardial Targeting With Contrast During Alcohol Septal Ablation

Paul Sorajja, MD

A 74-year-old woman with symptomatic, severe obstructive hypertrophic cardiomyopathy was brought to the cardiac catheterization laboratory for alcohol septal ablation. A, The most proximal septal perforator artery is wired with a standard 0.014″ soft-tip guide wire (arrow), followed by placement and inflation of a 1.5-mm over-the-wire angioplasty balloon to 3 atm. The guidewire is then removed. B, Through the angioplasty balloon, echocardiographic contrast (Definity) is injected with simultaneous transthoracic echocardiography. Echocardiography demonstrates contrast enhancement of ventricular septal myocardium that is intimately involved in the creation of systolic anterior of the mitral valve and left ventricular outflow tract obstruction (arrow). C, With further imaging, however, there also is contrast enhancement of the inferomedial papillary muscle (arrow). D, Additional imaging demonstrates contrast enhancement of the entire inferomedial papillary muscle extending toward the left ventricular free wall (arrow). Given the potential for papillary muscle infarction, the alcohol septal ablation procedure was then aborted.

Ao, Ascending aorta; LA, left atrium; LV, left ventricle.

KEY POINTS

- Contrast echocardiography is essential for successful alcohol septal ablation. The use of contrast echocardiography reduces infarct size and helps to avoid infarction of untoward areas of the myocardium.
- The assessment with contrast echocardiography during alcohol ablation entails a comprehensive examination of not only the ventricular septum, but also the entire right and left ventricular chambers and the papillary muscles. Once contrast has been injected through the balloon catheter, the echocardiographic assessment should continue to be performed when the balloon catheter is being flushed (i.e., with alcohol or saline).
- Alcohol septal ablation should not be performed when there is contrast enhancement of portions of the ventricular septum not related to left ventricular outflow tract obstruction, or any time there is enhancement of the ventricular free walls or papillary muscles.

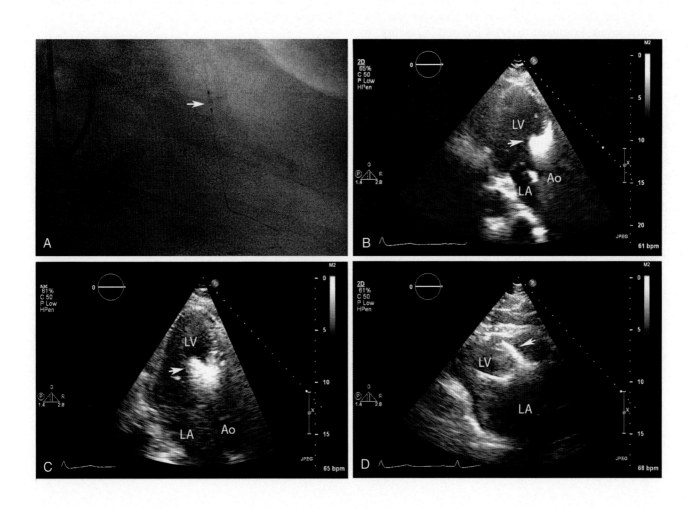

Case Selection for Alcohol Septal Ablation

Paul Sorajja, MD

Case selection is essential for procedural success with alcohol septal ablation for obstructive hypertrophic cardiomyopathy (HCM). In particular, these patients commonly have mitral valve (MV) abnormalities that may require additional surgical therapy. A–C, This patient was a 71-year-old woman with a 12-year history of HCM. Over the past year, she had developed severe exertional dyspnea that was refractory to medical therapy with β-receptor antagonists. Her transthoracic echocardiogram showed hypertrophy of the left ventricle (*) and systolic anterior motion (SAM) of the MV with septal-leaflet contact (arrowhead). However, on Doppler color-flow imaging, the direction of her mitral regurgitation (MR) was anterior (arrow), demonstrating that the MR is due to intrinsic valve disease and not secondary to SAM. Further imaging with transesophageal echocardiography confirmed the presence of a posterior leaflet flail segment. Thus, she was not a suitable candidate for alcohol septal ablation and underwent surgical repair. D–F, This patient was a 65-year-old woman with drug-refractory symptoms due to HCM. Transthoracic echocardiography demonstrated ventricular septal hypertrophy (*) and SAM with septal-leaflet contact

(arrowhead). On color-flow imaging, the direction of the MR jet is posterior (arrow) and thus typical for MR secondary to SAM. This patient then underwent successful alcohol septal ablation.

Ao, Ascending aorta; LA, left atrium; LV, left ventricle; RV, right ventricle.

KEY POINTS

- A careful, comprehensive examination for intrinsic MV disease is important in selecting patients with HCM for alcohol septal ablation.
- In patients with MR secondary to SAM, the direction of the MR jet is typically posterior-inferior. When the MR jet is not in this direction, one should be highly suspicious of intrinsic MV disease that may require additional surgical therapy.

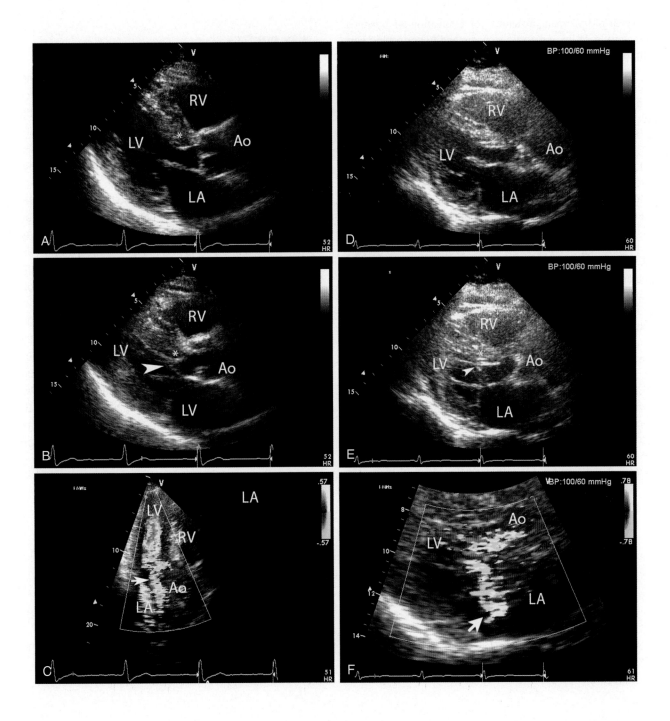

Assessment of Aortic Stenosis in Hypertrophic Cardiomyopathy

Paul Sorajja, MD

A 71-year-old woman presented for evaluation of dyspnea in the setting of known aortic stenosis and hypertrophic cardiomyopathy (HCM). A–D, On transthoracic echocardiography, there was ventricular septal hypertrophy (wall thickness, 2.1 cm), a calcified aortic valve, and mild systolic anterior of the mitral valve (arrowhead). On Doppler interrogation across the left ventricular outflow tract (LVOT) and aortic valve, the mean gradient was 33 mm Hg with a peak velocity of 3.7 m/s. There was uncertainty regarding the severity of her LVOT obstruction, as the Doppler signal across the aortic valve could not be differentiated from the underlying sub-aortic gradient. The patient was then referred for an invasive hemodynamic study in the cardiac catheterization laboratory. E, The invasive study was performed with transseptal puncture to allow positioning of a single end-hole, balloon wedge (BW) catheter in the left ventricular apex. This flotation catheter with no shaft side holes facilitates stable recording of apical pressures. A pigtail catheter is placed for ascending aorta (Ao) pressures. A multipurpose catheter allows sampling of pressures precisely at the left ventricular base, immediately beneath the aortic valve. F, Pressure recordings from the left ventricular apex, base, and Ao are shown. The mean gradient across the aortic valve is 32 mm Hg, and the peak gradient due to LVOT obstruction is 22 mm Hg. G, However, on the post-ectopic beat, a dynamic LVOT gradient of 105 mm Hg is evident, indicating that severe LVOT obstruction is present.

Ao, Ascending aorta; AV, aortic valve; BW, balloon wedge; LA, left atrium; LV, left ventricle; MP, multipurpose; PIG, pigtail catheter; RA, right atrium; RV, right ventricle; VS, ventricular septum.

KEY POINTS

- For patients with concomitant aortic stenosis and obstructive HCM, characterizing the severity of these two lesions with echocardiography can be challenging. This understanding is important, particularly when extended myectomy for HCM may be indicated, as this surgical procedure requires considerable technical expertise.

- An invasive hemodynamic study is highly accurate for determining the severity of aortic stenosis and LVOT obstruction due to HCM when they arise together, as sampling at multiple levels can be performed simultaneously at rest and with dynamic provocation in the cardiac catheterization laboratory.

- The transseptal approach offers a reliable method for pressure sampling with minimization of ectopy and potential for catheter entrapment. The side-arm of the transseptal sheath could also be used for left atrial pressures (not shown). An alternative method is to use two multipurpose catheters, with one of these catheters sampling the pressure at the left ventricular apex in place of the balloon wedge catheter.

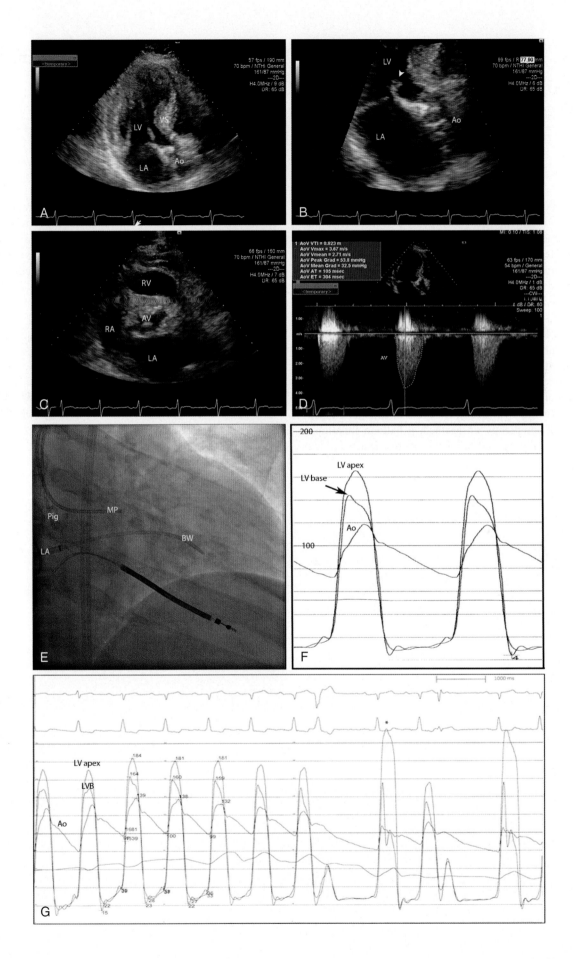

Transcatheter Left Ventricular Volume Reduction With Parachute in a Patient With Ischemic Cardiomyopathy

Adnan K. Chhatriwalla, MD

A 56-year-old woman with prior anterior wall myocardial infarction and ischemic cardiomyopathy presented with persistent dyspnea. Her functional status was consistent with New York Heart Association (NYHA) class III heart failure despite optimal medical therapy. A, Left ventriculography demonstrated an anteroapical aneurysm (arrowheads). Transcatheter left ventricular volume reduction was performed. B, The delivery sheath was advanced retrograde across the aortic valve to the left ventricle (LV) apex (white arrowhead) and an 85-mm Parachute device (Cardiokinetix, Menlo Park, CA) was advanced (black arrowhead) to the end of the sheath. C, The sheath is then retracted, with the foot of the device (black arrowhead) in contact with the LV apex, and as the device is unsheathed (white arrowhead), it begins to expand. D, After the device is completely unsheathed, a balloon inflation is performed to fully expand the device (arrowhead). E, Next, the balloon is deflated, and repeat ventriculography demonstrates exclusion of the LV apical aneurysm (arrowheads). F, Appropriate placement of the device at the LV apex can also be observed on echocardiography (arrowheads). Following the procedure, the patient's symptoms improved, consistent with NYHA class I functional status.

KEY POINTS

- Transcatheter LV volume reduction may help to restore LV geometry and improve symptoms and functional status.

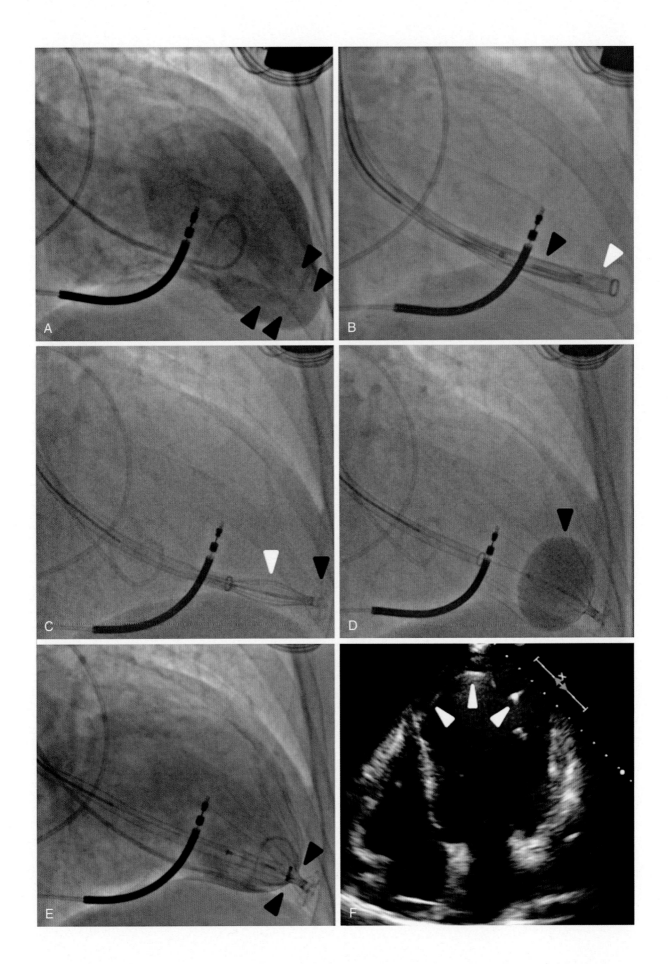

Congenital Abnormalities, Pseudoaneurysms, and Shunts

Closure of Patent Ductus Arteriosus

Ziyad Hijazi, MD, and Wail Alkashkari, MD

A 28-year-old woman was diagnosed with a heart murmur at 3.5 years of age. At 25 years of age, she was diagnosed with a large patent ductus arteriosus (PDA) when she became pregnant and suffered a miscarriage. After a subsequent, second miscarriage, the patient presented for further evaluation and management. Her major complaints were shortness of breath and fatigue. On examination, her blood pressure was 111/47 mm Hg, and there was a loud, machinery continuous murmur heard best at the left infraclavicular area. A, An echocardiogram revealed the presence of a large PDA, with left-to-right shunting and a transpulmonary gradient of 70 mm Hg (arrow). B, Her left ventricle had normal function (ejection fraction, 65%), but was enlarged with an end-diastolic dimension (LVEDD) of 71 mm on M-mode echocardiography. On cardiac catheterization, her Qp: Qs was 2:1, with a mean right pulmonary artery wedge pressure of 14 mm Hg, right pulmonary artery pressure of 61/34 mm Hg (mean, 47 mm Hg), and a descending aorta pressure of 135/52 mm Hg (mean, 80 mm Hg). These findings indicated that her pulmonary artery pressure was slightly under half-systemic, and the pulmonary vascular resistance was <5 Wood units. C, Using calibrations (arrow), angiography in the descending aorta revealed a large, type D PDA, measuring 11 mm at its narrowest diameter (arrows). In the right anterior oblique at 25 degrees, balloon sizing of the PDA with (D) full inflation (arrow) and (E) partial inflation (arrows) measured 12 mm. A 12-mm Amplatzer VSD occluder (St. Jude Medical, St. Paul, MN) was chosen to close the PDA due to the presence of pulmonary hypertension. F

and G, The device was delivered via an 8-Fr long delivery sheath (arrows). H, Repeat angiography confirmed satisfactory device positioning with the retention disks in place, with a mild residual shunt that was primarily through the device (arrow). Repeat hemodynamic assessment revealed that Qp : Qs ratio had dropped to 1.4:1. The pulmonary artery pressures also decreased to 36/20 mm Hg (mean, 28 mm Hg) in the setting of a descending aorta pressure of 144/70 mm Hg (mean, 96 mm Hg). The patient was discharged home the following day. At one-month follow-up, she reported improvement in her symptoms. Her examination was unremarkable. I, The transthoracic echocardiogram showed a completely occluded PDA (arrow), and her LVEDD had decreased to 55 mm.

KEY POINTS

- Untreated PDA is rare in the adult patient, and can cause left ventricular volume overload.
- An accurate hemodynamic assessment and assessment of operability is crucial prior to closure of a large PDA.
- When pulmonary hypertension is present, it is best to use an occluder that has two retention disks to minimize the risk of device embolization.

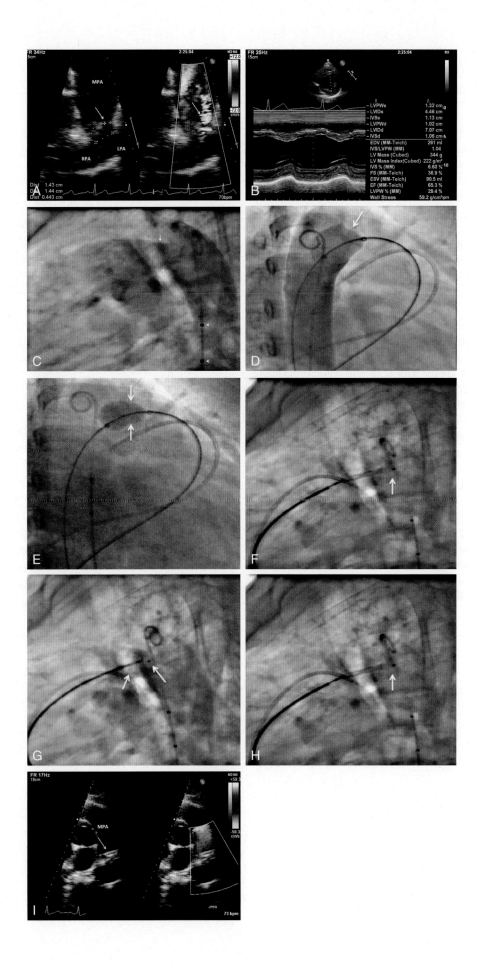

CONGENITAL ABNORMALITIES, PSEUDOANEURYSMS, AND SHUNTS

Complex PFO Closure Via Transseptal Puncture

Dominik M. Wiktor, MD, and John D. Carroll, MD

A 43-year-old man with a history of recurrent transient ischemic attacks and cryptogenic stroke on medical therapy was found to have a patent foramen ovale (PFO) by transthoracic echocardiography, and was referred for percutaneous PFO closure. A, He underwent preprocedural transesophageal echocardiogram that demonstrated a PFO with a bidirectional shunt (white arrow), a long tunnel (red arrow), suggesting that the tunnel may be noncompliant due to the thicker and brighter appearance of the septum primum. The defect was crossed, and a 20-mm Gore HELEX (W.L. Gore & Assoc., Tempe, AZ) was deployed; however, the device did not conform well and was removed. B, Next, a 30-mm Gore HELEX was deployed; however, splaying of the discs suggested a long, noncompliant tunnel, and the device was removed. C, Balloon sizing with a 30-mm × 4-cm NuMED PTS balloon (NuMed, Hopkinton, NY) was performed, and the waist on the balloon confirmed a long, noncompliant tunnel. D, The site of transseptal puncture of the septum primum was planned to be close to the right atrial entry to the PFO (white arrow). After puncture, the transseptal sheath was exchanged for a 10-Fr, 80-cm Arrow-Flex sheath. A 30-mm Gore HELEX device was redeployed across the transseptal puncture site. E, The device discs were now flat by X-ray and device locking was confirmed. F, Predischarge transthoracic echocardiography in the subcostal view confirmed that both discs remained well apposed to both sides of the septum (left panel) with no residual shunting by color Doppler (right panel).

LA, Left atrium; RA, right atrium.

KEY POINTS

- The majority of PFO closures can be performed with standard crossing and device occlusion techniques using the PFO itself. However, a subset of defects will require advanced techniques, such as transseptal puncture to achieve closure.
- Long, rigid PFO tunnels (usually >12 mm in length) are the most common reason why transseptal puncture may be required. The rigid tunnel "pulls" the atrial discs into the defect, preventing the disc from flattening with variable degrees of residual shunting.
- Balloon sizing is helpful to outline the tunnel length, morphology, and compliance.
- If transseptal puncture is needed, the septum primum puncture should be located very close to the PFO inlet to ensure the left atrial disc of the device will be long enough to cover the outlet of the tunnel. Positioning close to the right atrial disc is also important for apposing the primum and secundum to close the inlet of the tunnel.
- There may still be an increased rate of residual shunting in PFOs closed via transseptal puncture. Optimizing the location of the transseptal puncture and the size of the closure device are key technical considerations.
- Echocardiography with either intracardiac or transesophageal imaging is needed to ensure that a residual leak does not exist along the crescentic PFO margins.

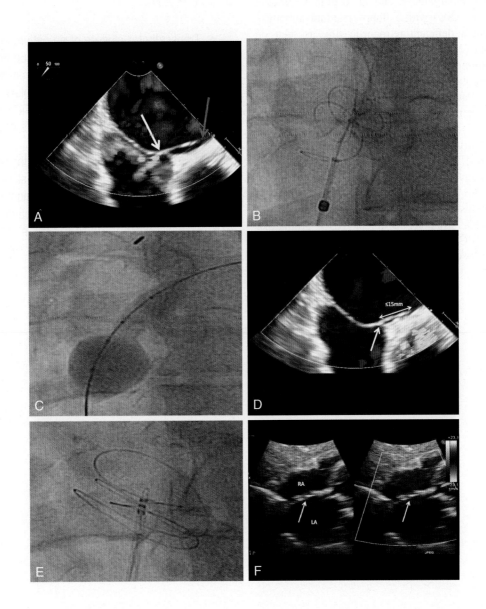

Clockwise Maneuver for ASD Closure

Matthew J. Price, MD

A 48-year-old man presented with dyspnea on exertion, right-sided cardiac enlargement, and an ostium secundum atrial septal defect (ASD) with a floppy residual interatrial septum (IAS) and a deficient retroaortic rim, as seen on (A) 2-dimensional (2-D) transesophageal echocardiography (TEE) and (B) 3-dimensional (3-D) TEE. The initial attempt using a 28-mm Amplatzer Septal Occluder (ASO) device (St. Jude Medical, St. Paul, MN) was unsuccessful because (C) the angle formed by the delivery sheath and the plane of the IAS was too narrow, resulting in (D) the left atrial disc slipping into the right atrium at the site of the deficient retroaortic rim (double arrows). E and F, Aggressive counterclockwise rotation of the delivery sheath established an orthogonal approach to the IAS resulting in (G and H) stable position and successful occlusion with an ASO 30-mm device.

Ao, Aorta; ASD, atrial septal defect; ASO, Amplatzer Septal Occluder; IVC, inferior venae cavae; LA, left atrium; RA, right atrium; SVC, superior venae cavae.

KEY POINTS

- Transcatheter closure of an ostium secundum ASD with a deficient retroaortic rim can be challenging, as the left atrial side of the occluder device will often slip into the RA during deployment. This can occur when the orientation of the delivery sheath within the left atrium (LA) is not sufficient orthogonal to the plane of the IAS.
- Aggressive clockwise rotation of the standard delivery sheath can orient the distal sheath perpendicular to the plane of the IAS, which will then align the left atrial disc of the device parallel to the ASD. This will allow the disc to "catch" the aorta when the system is withdrawn to the IAS and the right atrial disc is deployed.

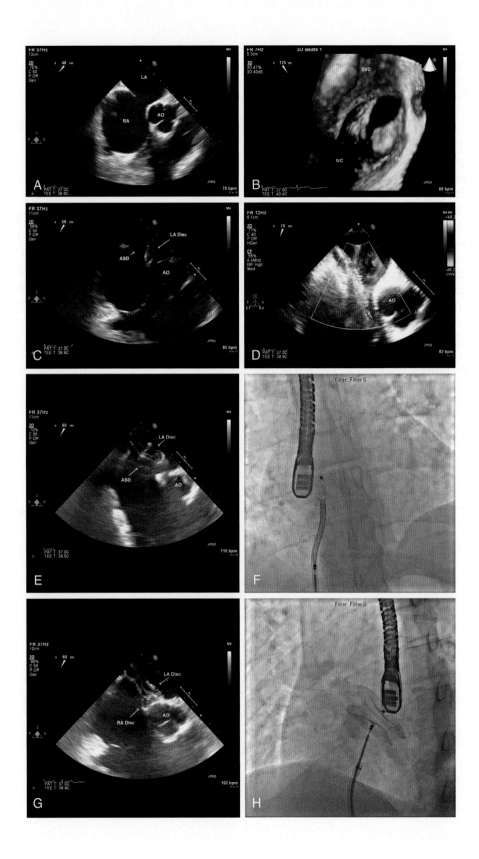

Sizing Balloon to Facilitate ASD Closure

Matthew J. Price, MD

A 37-year-old woman presented with dyspnea on exertion, right-sided cardiac enlargement, and a large ostium secundum ASD with a deficient retroaortic rim, as seen on (A) 2-D TEE and (B) 3-D TEE. C, Initial attempt with a 26-mm ASO device failed as the left atrial disk fell into the RA at the site of the deficient aortic rim (arrow). D and E, A sizing balloon catheter was advanced alongside the delivery sheath through a second venous access, and inflated slightly so that it would push and orient the axis of the left atrial disc parallel to the plane of the IAS (or the sheath more orthogonal to the IAS). F, With this approach, the device was deployed in a stable and successful fashion.

Ao, Aorta; ASD, atrial septal defect; ASO, Amplatzer Septal Occluder; IVC, inferior venae cavae; LA, left atrium; RA, right atrium; SVC, superior venae cavae.

KEY POINTS

1. In patient in need of ASD closure and with deficient rims, clockwise rotation may not be sufficient.
2. In these cases, a sizing balloon catheter can be advanced into the LA through a second venous sheath. The catheter is manipulated alongside the left atrial disc to deflect it away from the aorta and orient it parallel to the IAS as the sheath is withdrawn and the right atrial disc is deployed.

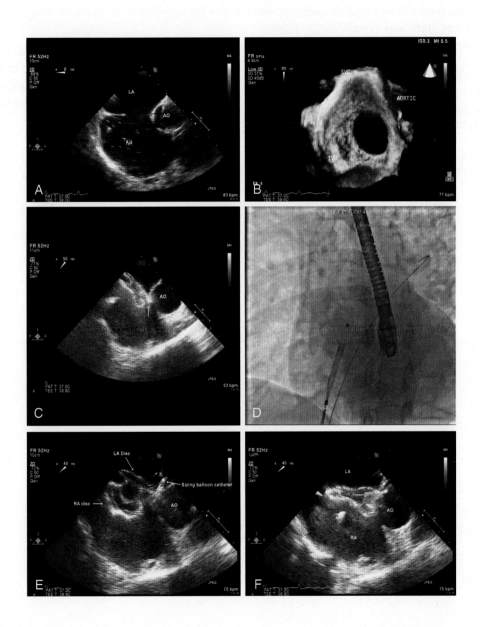

Curve of Distal Sheath and Closure of ASD With Deficient Rim
Matthew J. Price, MD

A 34-year-old woman presented with right-sided cardiac enlargement, a Qp : Qs ratio of 1.9 : 1, and an ostium secundum ASD with deficient aortic rim as seen on (A) intracardiac echocardiography (ICE). B, A 20-mm ASO device was advanced through a 10-Fr Swartz Left (SL)-2 sheath, the distal shape of which aligns the axis of the left atrial disk parallel to the IAS. C and D, This maneuver allowed the device to be implanted in a single attempt in an optimal and stable position without the need for repositioning.

Ao, Aorta; ASD, atrial septal defect; ASO, Amplatzer Septal Occluder; IVC, inferior venae cavae; LA, left atrium; RA, right atrium; SVC, superior venae cavae.

KEY POINTS

For patients with deficient rims and in need of ASD closure, the device can be dlievered through a sheath with a different distal curve that positions the device parallel to the IAS, cu as an SL-2 or Hausdorf sheath.

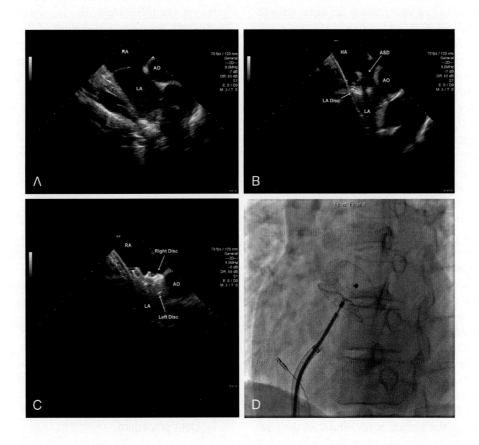

Closure of Patent Foramen Ovale Using a Cardioform Septal Occluder

Mario Gössl, MD, PhD

A 49-year-old man suffered an acute cerebrovascular event with acute onset of right-hand weakness. Magnetic resonance imaging showed multiple, presumably embolic infarctions in the distribution of the left middle cranial artery, but no intracranial or extracranial artery stenoses. Further comprehensive evaluation, including examination for atrial arrhythmias and coagulopathy, led to the diagnosis of cryptogenic stroke due to patent foramen ovale (PFO). A, Closure of his PFO using a Gore Cardioform Septal Occluder device (Gore, Flagstaff, AZ) was undertaken. The procedure was performed with conscious sedation using intracardiac echocardiography (ICE) imaging. After obtaining access to the right femoral vein with an 11-Fr sheath for device delivery, and a 30-cm long, 9-Fr Cook sheath for ICE imaging in the left femoral vein, anticoagulation with intravenous heparin was initiated (goal range, 250–300 sec). B, ICE image of the interatrial septum (*) demonstrated the PFO with bidirectional shunting (arrow). The limbus had an acceptable thickness, without a redundant septum and no significant tunnel. Hence, a 25-mm Gore Cardioform Septal Occluder device was chosen. C, The PFO was crossed with a straight, 0.038″ guidewire (*) and a 6-Fr multipurpose coronary catheter. The wire is then exchanged for a 0.035″ Amplatzer extra-stiff exchange-length wire with a self-made left atrial curve. Using the Amplatzer wire for support, the Gore Cardioform Septal Occluder delivery system is advanced monorail into the left atrium, followed by removal of the wire. D and E, The left atrial disc (*) is formed by moving the slider of the (J) Gore Cardioform Septal Occluder handle to the left. The center eyelet is seen exiting the delivery catheter (arrow) until a flat left disc is formed. F and G, Subsequently, the system is pulled back until resistance at the septum is felt, and then the right atrial disc is formed by moving the slider further to the left

(*). Once the operator is satisfied with the position on ICE imaging, the device is locked for a tension-free assessment, whereby the right hand holds the handle in place and the left hand squeezes and moves the Occluder Lock to the right. The Occluder remains tethered to the delivery system by the Retrieval Cord. Subsequently, the retrieval cord is removed by flipping, twisting, and pulling of the retrieval cord lock. H and I, Fluoroscopic and ICE imaging shows the released Gore Cardioform Septal Occluder device (*), confirming the Occluder is locked and demonstrating excellent anatomical position without residual shunting.

LA, Left atrium; RA, right atrium; SVC, superior vena cava.

KEY POINTS

- Closure of PFO for cryptogenic stroke is an FDA-approved procedure in the United States.
- ICE imaging for PFO closure facilitates conscious sedation for the procedure.
- The Gore Cardioform Septal Occluder is currently available in 15-, 20-, 25-, and 30-mm diameters, with the recommended defect size to Cardioform ratio being >1:1.75.
- The conformable nature of the Gore Cardioform Septal Occluder (ePTFE membrane applied to a five-wire frame with a platinum core nitinol wire) and ease of deployment permits a safe and efficient procedure.

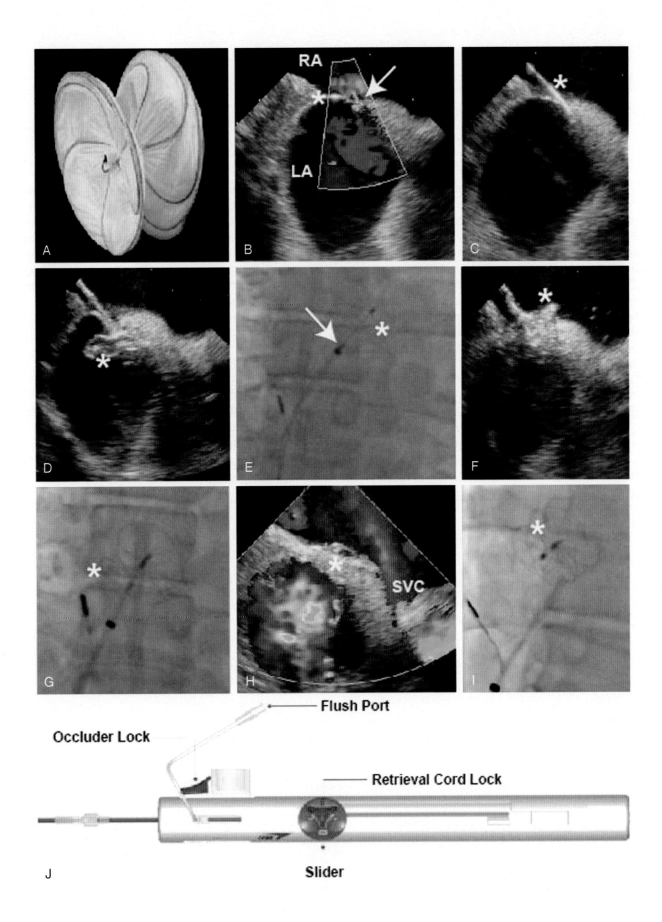

RA

LA

A

B

C

D

E

F

G

H

SVC

I

Flush Port

Occluder Lock

Retrieval Cord Lock

Slider

J

Transcatheter Open-Cell Stent Implantation for Treatment of Native Coarctation of the Aorta

Jason H. Anderson, MD, and Allison K. Cabalka, MD

A 36-year-old man with systemic hypertension due to native coarctation of the aorta presented for catheter-based therapy. A femoral arterial approach was utilized with placement of two Perclose Proglide devices (Abbott, Chicago, IL). Hemodynamic evaluation documented a 48-mm Hg, peak-to-peak systolic gradient. Three-dimensional rotational angiography (3DRA) was performed with ascending aorta injection (Omnipaque 50 cc, injected at 8 cc/sec under RV pacing at 200 bpm), demonstrating (A) a transverse arch diameter of 22 mm (arrow), (B) minimum coarctation diameter of 8 × 10 mm (arrow), and post-stenotic dilatation of the descending thoracic aorta to 25 mm. A 0.035″ Amplatz Super-Stiff Exchange wire (Medtronic, Minneapolis, MN) was placed across the coarctation segment, and the introducer was upsized to a 12-Fr Mullins sheath (Medtronic, Minneapolis, MN). C, A 36-mm Intrastent LD Max (ev3 Endovascular Inc, Plymouth, MN) bare metal stent was mounted on an 18-mm × 4-cm BIB balloon (B. Braun Medical Inc., Bethlehem, PA) (arrow) and deployed under 3DRA/fluoroscopy overlay. Proximal (D) and distal flaring of the stent was performed with a 22-mm × 4-cm Tyshak balloon (B. Braun Medical Inc.) (arrow). E, Flaring into the right subclavian artery was performed with a 14-mm × 3-cm Z-med II balloon (B. Braun Medical Inc.) (arrow). F, Postimplantation 3DRA demonstrated stent apposition with the vessel wall with no contrast extravasation or compromised blood flow into the brachiocephalic vessels (arrow). No residual peak-to-peak systolic gradient was present.

KEY POINTS

- Open-cell stents demonstrate improved conformity to the transverse aortic arch. Each cell can be separately dilated to prevent brachiocephalic jailing.
- Covered stents are indicated for cases with concomitant aortic aneurysm or high risk for vascular complications.

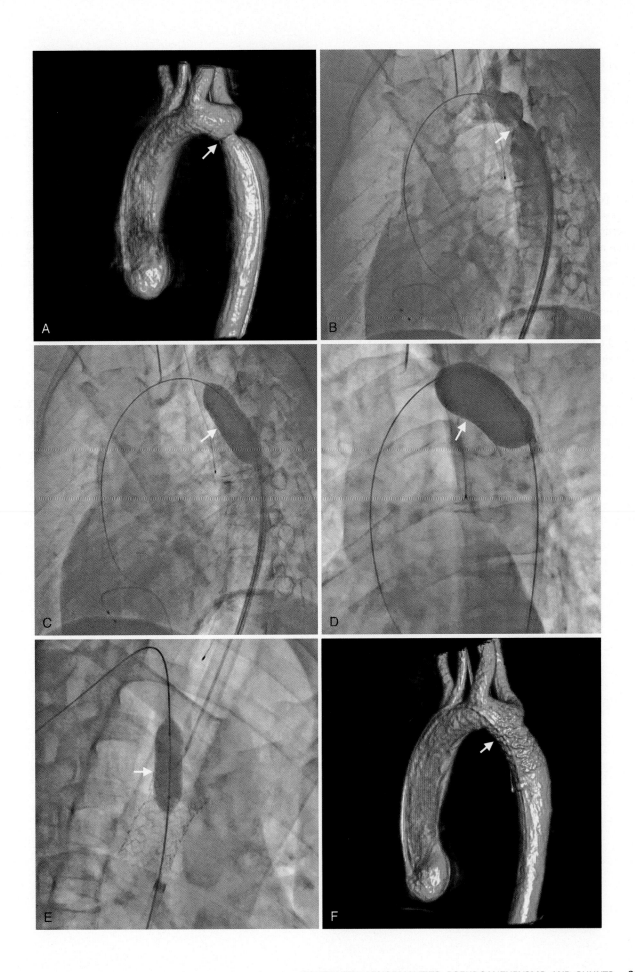

Transcatheter Device Closure of a Post Myocardial Infarction Ventricular Septal Defect

Jason H. Anderson, MD, Paul Sorajja, MD, and Allison K. Cabalka, MD

An 81-year-old woman presented with exertional dyspnea due to a post myocardial infarction ventricular septal defect, in the setting of a prior anterior myocardial infarction. Femoral arterial and right internal jugular venous access was utilized. A, Ventriculography demonstrated a large, apical septal rupture with multiple channels entering the right ventricle (arrows). B, Transesophageal echocardiography documented a 14-mm entry point from the left ventricle (arrows). A 6-Fr Amplatz left guide catheter allowed for passage of a 0.035″ Angled Glidewire (Terumo Medial Corp., Somerset, NJ) into the main pulmonary artery. C, The wire was snared from the right internal jugular vein to form an arteriovenous rail (arrow). The guide was advanced to the right atrium allowing for placement of a second guidewire, a 0.035″ Amplatzer "noodlewire" guidewire (St. Jude Medical, St. Paul, MN), forming an additional arteriovenous rail. D, A 9-Fr Amplatzer TorqVue Delivery System (St. Jude Medical) was advanced over the noodlewire and placed in the left ventricular apex (arrow). E, An 18-mm Amplatzer Muscular ventricular septal defect (VSD) Occluder (St. Jude Medical) was deployed across the VSD (arrow). The glidewire was removed. F, Left ventricular angiography was repeated showing a mild residual left-to-right shunt and stable device position. G and H, The device was successfully deployed. Resolution of her symptoms was ascertained with a trivial, hemodynamically insignificant residual shunt present on routine follow-up, with normal left atrial and left ventricular size.

LV, Left ventricle; RV, right ventricle.

KEY POINTS

- Sheath kinking can complicate device delivery and may necessitate re-creation of an arteriovenous guidewire rail.
- If possible, delaying device implantation for a VSD for 3 to 4 weeks after an infarction is advisable, improving fibrosis of the myocardium for anchoring of the closure device.

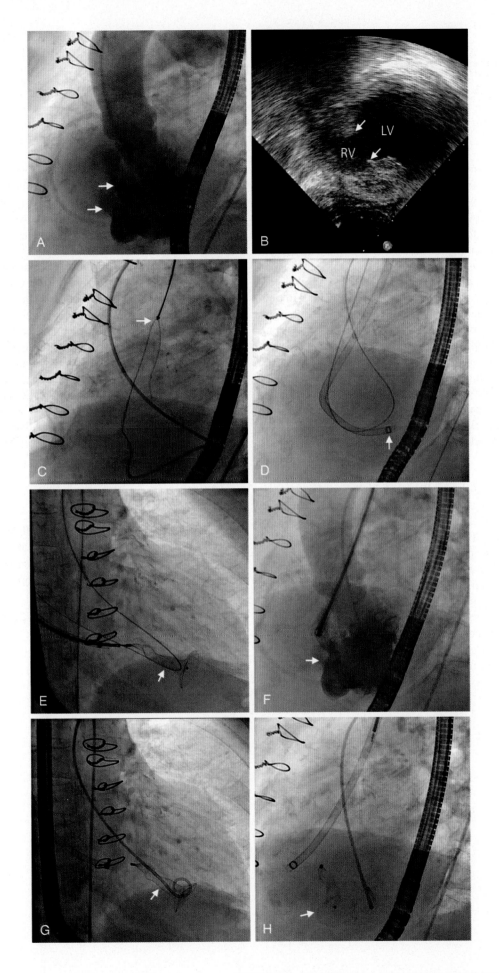

Post-Surgical Ventricular Septal Defect Therapy

Paul Sorajja, MD, Mario Gössl, MD, Marcus Burns, DNP, and Richard Y. Bae, MD

A 70-year-old man presented with cardiogenic shock, immediately after septal myectomy and surgical aortic valve replacement with a 27-mm Edwards Magna prosthesis (Edwards Lifesciences, Irvine, CA). At re-operation, the lesion was not felt to be repairable, and the patient was placed on extracorporeal membrane oxygenation (ECMO). A, On transesophageal echocardiography (TEE), there was a large ventricular septal defect (VSD) at the base of the heart (arrowhead), with (B) severe intracardiac shunting (arrowhead). The defect was initially crossed from the right ventricle (RV) via right internal jugular venous access, but delivery sheaths could not be passed and the wire could not be advanced out the aortic prosthesis for snaring. C, The aortic prosthesis was then crossed retrograde with an Amplatz left catheter, followed by exchange for a Judkins right coronary catheter (JR) and passage of a glidewire (W) from the left ventricle into the RV (arrowhead). D, The wire was placed in the pulmonary artery, where it was snared with a 15-mm gooseneck that had been advanced from the right internal jugular vein (arrowhead). E, The wire was then exteriorized as a venoarterial rail (arrowheads). Initially, a 9-Fr delivery sheath was used to place an 18-mm Amplatzer VSD occluder (St. Jude Medical, St. Paul, MN), but there was significant residual shunting. Following removal of this occluder, a 12-Fr DrySeal sheath (W.L. Gore & Associates, Flagstaff, AZ) was placed over the glidewire in the internal jugular vein. F, The 18-mm VSD occluder was then placed in the defect again (arrow) using the 9-Fr delivery catheter (arrowhead). The 12-Fr DrySeal would not accommodate both the delivery cable of the occluder and an 8-Fr delivery sheath, so (G) the delivery sheath was then placed retrograde across the aortic valve (arrow), with the delivery cable (DC) still attached to the 18-mm device (arrowhead). A 16-mm VSD occluder was then extruded (H) partially (arrow) and then (I) fully (arrowheads). J, Fluoroscopy showed stable final positioning of the 18-mm device (arrows) and the 16-mm device (arrowheads). K, Post-deployment TEE shows the devices in place (arrowhead). L, There was mild-moderate residual shunting, mainly through the device occluders (arrowhead). Additional imaging also revealed a flail tricuspid leaflet, with no change in regurgitation, related to catheter manipulation (not shown). The patient's tissue perfusion improved. However, ECMO weaning led to onset of severe left ventricular outflow tract obstruction from systolic anterior motion of the mitral valve and hemodynamic instability. The patient subsequently underwent successful surgery with repeat myectomy, tricuspid valve replacement, and repair of the VSD.

AV, Aortic valve prosthesis; DC, delivery cable; LA, left atrium; LV, left ventricle; RV, right ventricle; W, guidewire.

KEY POINTS

- Transcatheter repair of VSDs can be challenging to the eccentric nature of these lesions. Multiple occluders may be considered for closure.
- Entanglement and injury in the chordal apparatus is a complication of VSD closure.
- Use of a rail provides support for delivery catheter passed antegrade and retrograde, and also serves as an anchor to minimize wire re-crossing.

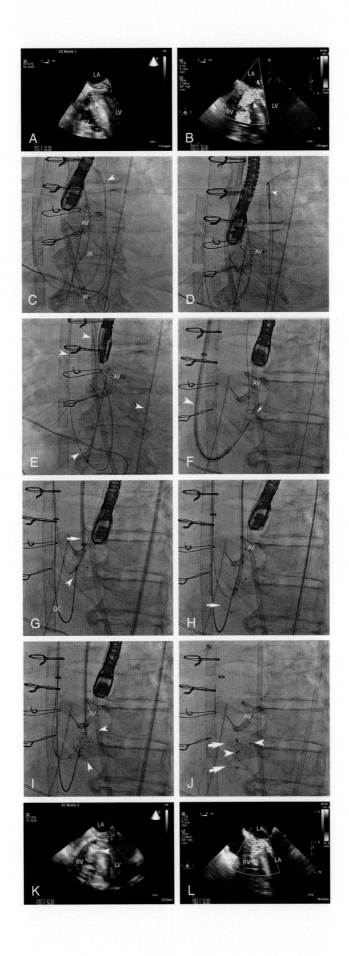

CONGENITAL ABNORMALITIES, PSEUDOANEURYSMS, AND SHUNTS 241

Ventricular Septal Defect Closure

Ziyad Hijazi, and Wail Alkashkari

A 37-year-old woman with a history of prior surgical repair for tetralogy of Fallot and recent transcatheter pulmonary homograft repair presented for transcatheter closure of a ventricular septal defect (VSD). Angiography in the left ventricle (LV), prior to placement of the pulmonary valve, was performed in biplane (25 degrees right anterior oblique and 60 degrees left anterior oblique/15 degrees cranial). This angiogram revealed the presence of a moderate sized peri-membranous VSD measuring approximately 8 to 10 mm (A, arrow). Following pulmonary valve deployment, the VSD was crossed from the LV using a 5-Fr Judkins catheter with a 0.035″ Terumo angled glidewire. The wire was snared in the main pulmonary artery and exteriorized through the right femoral vein. Over this wire, a 9-Fr delivery sheath was inserted and positioned in the ascending aorta. A 12-mm Amplatzer Muscular VSD occluder (St. Jude Medical, St. Paul, MN) was introduced into the sheath. The left ventricular disc was partially deployed in the ascending aorta (B, arrow). The entire assembly (sheath/device) was withdrawn until the sheath was under the aortic valve, where the entire left disc was deployed. Transesophageal echocardiography (TEE) and left ventricular angiography revealed good position of the disc away from the aortic valve (C, arrow). The connecting waist was then deployed in the VSD, followed by deployment of the right ventricular disc in the right ventricle (D, arrow). The right ventricular disc assumed a "cobra shape." The device was recaptured multiple times, but the abnormal shape remained, likely due to the tension from the cable. After confirmation with TEE and cine-angiography that the position was good, the device was released. Immediately, the right ventricular disc assumed its normal shape. Final left ventricular angiography revealed excellent device position (arrow) and minimal residual shunt (E). The catheters were removed and hemostasis in the vein was achieved using figure-of-eight stitch and manual compression for the left femoral artery. A week later, repeat TTE revealed good device position and no residual shunt (F and G, arrows).

LA, Left atrium; LV, left ventricle; RV, right ventricle.

KEY POINTS

- Residual VSD after surgical repair of tetralogy of Fallot is common and can be treated with transcatheter closure.
- Care should be undertaken to ensure the VSD is ≥2 mm away from the aortic valve when Amplatzer muscular VSD occluders are utilized.
- Imaging with echocardiography should be performed to ensure no interference with aortic valve function.

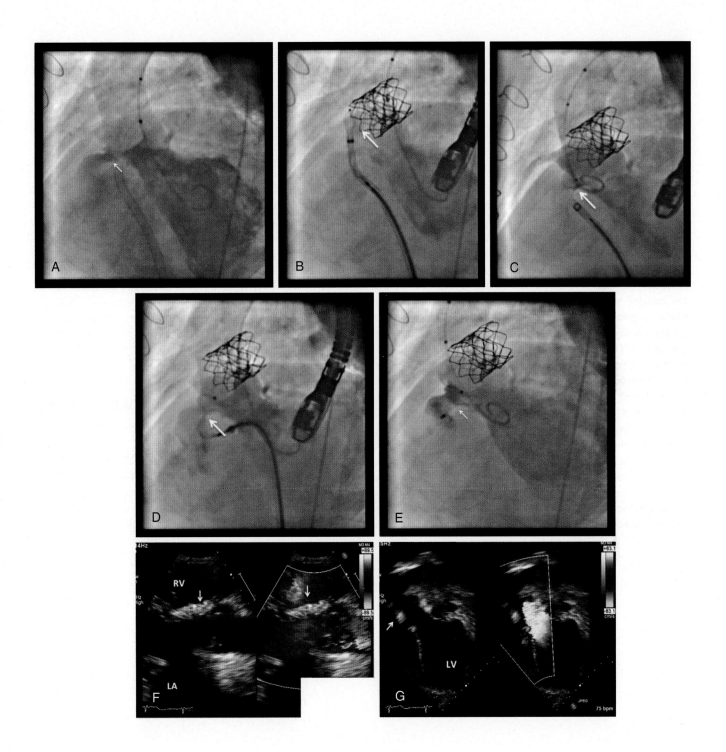

Percutaneous Closure of Postinfarction Ventricular Septal Defect

O. Alsanjari, A. Myat, and David Hildick-Smith, MD, FRCP

A 66-year-old woman was admitted with an inferior ST-elevation myocardial infarction complicated by a ventricular septal defect (VSD). Transesophageal echocardiography (TEE) demonstrated a large basal VSD with hemodynamically-significant, left-to-right shunting (A and B). The defect was evident on fluoroscopy during left ventriculography (C, arrow). The patient was referred for percutaneous closure.

Under general anesthesia and with TEE, the defect was crossed with a pigtail catheter from the right femoral artery. A guidewire (Terumo, Somerset, NJ) was passed to the pulmonary artery, and deliberately prolapsed into the right atrium (RA). The wire was advanced from the RA to the inferior vena cava, where it was snared. The snare was then advanced to the pigtail catheter. The guidewire was removed, and an Amplatzer Noodle wire (St. Jude Medical, St. Paul, MN) passed through the pigtail, snared, and exteriorized. Using the rail, a 10-Fr guide was used to deliver a 24-mm Amplatzer postinfarction ventricular septal occluder device (St. Jude Medical, St. Paul, MN; D–F). The device fit well on the left ventricular side of the defect, but formed a cobra-type shape on the right ventricular side. After deliberation, the device was released in this configuration (G). There was some residual flow across the defect but we elected to permit this result, with the expectation that the device shape would mold itself and achieve satisfactory closure. Subsequent echocardiography (H) on postoperative day 1 and at 1 week showed that the deformation of the right ventricular disk remained, but repeat echocardiography at 1 month demonstrated reshaping of the right ventricular disc with concomitant full closure of the defect.

AV, Aortic valve; LA, left atrium; LV, left ventricle; MV, mitral valve; RA, right atrium; RV, right ventricle; VSD, ventricular septal defect.

KEY POINTS

- For percutaneous closure of acute VSD, upsize the device occluder by at least 100% relative to the defect.
- The left ventricular disc should be well formed, but the shape of the right ventricular disc may be irregular and reshape over several weeks after placement.

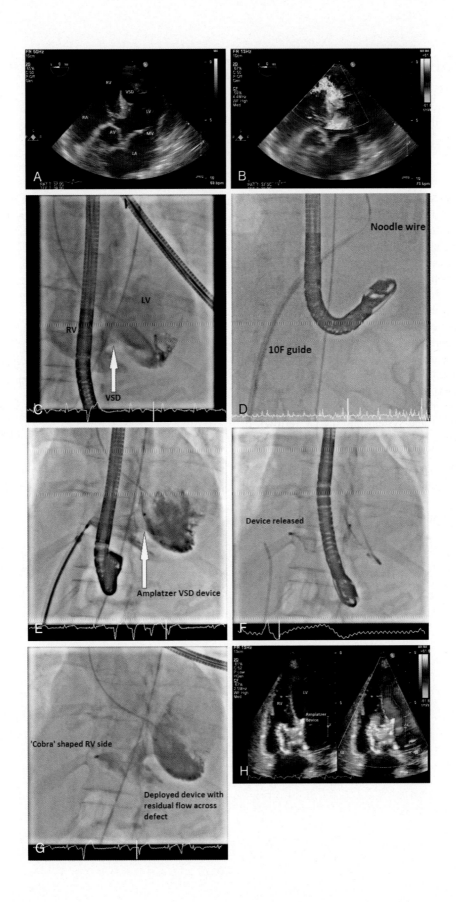

Patent Foramen Ovale Closure From the Right Internal Jugular Vein

Anil Poulose, MD, and Paul Sorajja, MD

A 47-year-old woman with a history of inferior vena cava occlusion was referred for closure of a patent foramen ovale (PFO) in the setting of cryptogenic stroke. A, From the right internal jugular vein, a 5-Fr multipurpose catheter (arrow) and glidewire (arrowhead) are used to cross the PFO with fluoroscopic and echocardiographic guidance. B, Passage of an 8-Fr delivery catheter is unsuccessful due to prolapse of the wire (arrowhead) into the left ventricle (LV) with antegrade movement. C, Using the same 8-Fr delivery catheter (arrow), a 6-Fr Judkins right coronary catheter (arrowhead) is used to pass a soft coronary guidewire, followed by further advancement of the coronary catheter into the left atrium to exchange for a stiff wire. D, Despite placement of the stiff wire in the left atrium, advancement of the delivery catheter still leads to prolapse of the wires and system into the LV (arrow). E, An 8.5-Fr, small-curve, steerable Agilis catheter (SGC) (St. Jude Medical, St. Paul, MN) is used to position an Amplatz Super Stiff wire in the left atrium (arrowhead). F, With articulation, the steerable catheter can be advanced into the left atrium over the stiff wire (arrowhead). G, The wire is then removed, leaving the catheter in the left atrium (arrowhead).

H, The left atrial disc of a 25-mm Cribriform occluder (St. Jude Medical, St. Paul, MN) is deployed (arrowhead). I, The right atrial disc is extruded (arrow). J, Final deployment of the device occluder (arrowhead).

SGC, Steerable guide catheter.

KEY POINTS

- Passage of catheters from the superior veins through a PFO can be challenging due to the acute angulation of the atrial septum.
- In these scenarios, use of a steerable catheter enhances tracking over the guidewire for safe passage into the left atrium.
- The bore of these steerable catheters is frequently large enough for delivery of device occluders (i.e., >8-Fr).

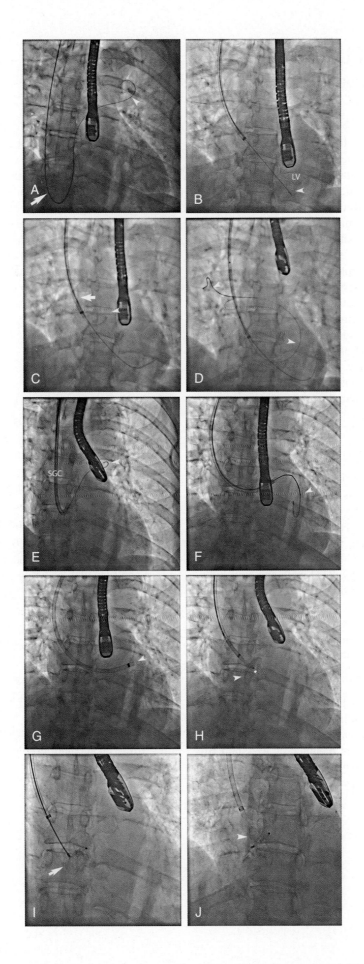

Pulmonary Homograft Therapy

Wail Alkashkari, MD, Gurdeep Mann, MD, and Ziyad M. Hijazi, MD

A 37-year-old woman with tetralogy of Fallot and absent pulmonary valve underwent her first surgical repair at 25 years of age, consisting of transannular patch repair and closure of a ventricular septal defect (VSD). Two years later, due to severe pulmonary insufficiency and residual VSD, she underwent placement of a 22-mm Contegra graft placement between the right ventricle and pulmonary artery. She did well until having symptoms of shortness of breath over the past year. At an outside institution, she was found to have severe obstruction in the Contegra graft and a residual VSD; balloon angioplasty of the Contegra graft was unsuccessful. Her transthoracic echocardiogram revealed a peak gradient of 80 mm Hg in the graft. Additional imaging revealed a moderate-sized residual VSD at the superior margin of the patch. Computed tomography angiography measured the narrowest diameter of the Contegra graft obstruction to be 13 mm in the oblique sagittal and paraxial views (arrows, A and B). Three-dimensional volume rendered images showed the obstructed conduit (arrows, C and D) and giant pulmonary arteries.

Cardiac catheterization was performed using a 16-Fr sheath in the right femoral vein and a 5-Fr sheath in the left femoral artery. The Qp:Qs ratio was 1.9:1 due to the residual VSD. Her pulmonary artery pressure was normal (22/9 mm Hg; mean, 17 mm Hg). The gradient across the Contegra graft was 43 mm Hg with an RV:DAO (descending aorta) pressure ratio of 0.74:1. Initial angiography in the Contegra graft revealed hugely dilated main and branch pulmonary arteries. The narrowest diameter was confirmed to be 13 mm (arrows, E and F).

Balloon inflation and simultaneous ascending aorta angiography was performed to examine the proximity of the coronary arteries to the right ventricle outflow tract (RVOT), demonstrating the distance to be safe (>10 mm) (arrows, G and H).

After positioning a 0.035″ Lunderquist wire in the left pulmonary artery, a 14-Fr Mullins Cook sheath was placed in the main pulmonary artery above the Contegra graft (I–L). A 39-mm long-covered CP stent mounted on a 22-mm BIB (balloon-in-balloon) was deployed in the Contegra graft to create a landing zone. Repeat angiography in the main pulmonary artery revealed excellent stent position and no complications.

The long Mullins sheath was removed, keeping the Lunderquist wire in position. A 16-Fr Edwards e-sheath was inserted in the right femoral vein. A 23-mm Edwards Sapien XT valve (Edwards Lifesciences, Irvine, CA) was placed in the middle of the CP stent (M and N). Repeat hemodynamic assessment revealed gradient of 12 mm Hg and the RV:DAO pressure ratio of 0.38:1. Final angiography revealed no pulmonary insufficiency and no complications (O and P).

Ao, Ascending aorta; LA, left atrium; LPA, left pulmonary artery; LV, left ventricle; RPA, right pulmonary artery; RV, right ventricle.

KEY POINTS

- Assessment of the proximity of the coronary arteries to the RVOT during pulmonary valve implantation is crucial. Approximately 5% of patients have abnormal origin of the coronary arteries, rendering them ineligible for transcatheter pulmonary valve replacement (tPVR).
- Placement of a landing zone is not an absolute requirement for therapy with the Edwards Sapien valve, but, due to the short height of the prosthesis, can help with accurate positioning.
- The use of covered stents is not an absolute requirement. However, when performing tPVR, immediate access to covered stents/grafts for bailout situations is needed in the event of homograft dissection or rupture.
- Use of ultra-stiff wires is very important in tPVR. Positioning of the wire in the left pulmonary artery is helpful.
- Slow inflation of the valve prosthesis allows accurate positioning of the valve inside the landing zone.

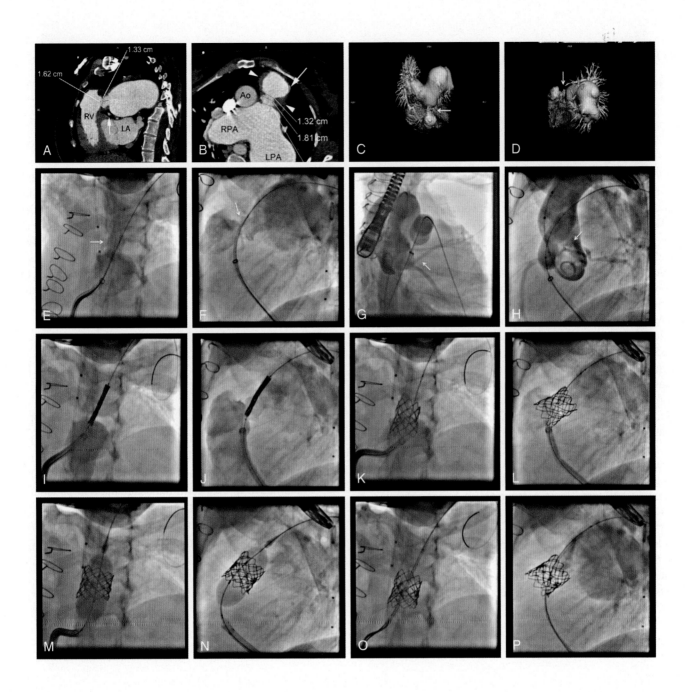

Left Atrial Appendage Closure With Watchman

Jay Thakkar, MD, and Jacqueline Saw, MD

A 79-year-old man with persistent non-valvular atrial fibrillation had spontaneous subarachnoid bleeding while on theraputic warfarin, and subsequently recovered functionally. His CHADS2 score was 4 and CHADS-Vasc score was 5, and he was referred for left atrial appendage (LAA) closure. A, and (B) Baseline imaging were performed to exclude LAA thrombus and assess LAA anatomy. Preprocedural cardiac computed tomography angiography (CCTA) showed a challenging superior-anteriorly directed (retroflex) chicken-wing LAA anatomy. C, For the Watchman device (Boston Scientific, Natick, MA), the widest LAA ostium at 0, 45, 90 and 135 degrees, and LAA depth were measured on transesophageal echocardiogram (TEE), and the maximum diameter was 27.8 mm and depth was 29 mm. The procedure was performed under general anesthesia and TEE guidance. Right femoral venous access was obtained. Transseptal puncture was performed with an SL1 sheath and BRK-XS needle in an inferoposterior position of the fossa ovalis, to enable coaxial sheath access into the retroflex LAA. Activated clotting time (ACT) was maintained >250 s and mean left atrial pressure >12 mm Hg (for accurate LAA measurments). A 14-Fr anterior-curve sheath was preplanned based on CCTA for the retroflex LAA, and was advanced to the left upper pulmonary vein through a Super-Stiff Amplatz wire. D, A 6-Fr marker pigtail was then used to advance the sheath into the LAA and cineangiogram performed. E, The access sheath was advanced into LAA distally and counter-clocked to maintain anterior-superior direction. F, A 33-mm Watchman device was deployed in the proximal LAA, and tug test showed good anchoring. The PASS criteria were verified, with good position (P), anchor (A: stable on tug), (G) size (S: compression 8% to 20%), and (H) seal (S: peri-device leak <5 mm). (I) The device was released and final 3-dimensional TEE showed successful placement. The patient tolerated the procedure well and was discharged the following day after transthoracic echocardiogram.

KEY POINTS

- Percutaneous LAA occlusion can be performed safely (risk of major periprocedural complication <1.5% including ischemic stroke, pericardial tamponade, and device embolization), and is a feasible alternative to long-term anticoagulation in patients with non-valvular atrial fibrillation.
- CCTA is a useful complimentary imaging modality to TEE for preprocedural planning, especially for complex anatomy.
- PASS criteria should be achieved for implantation.

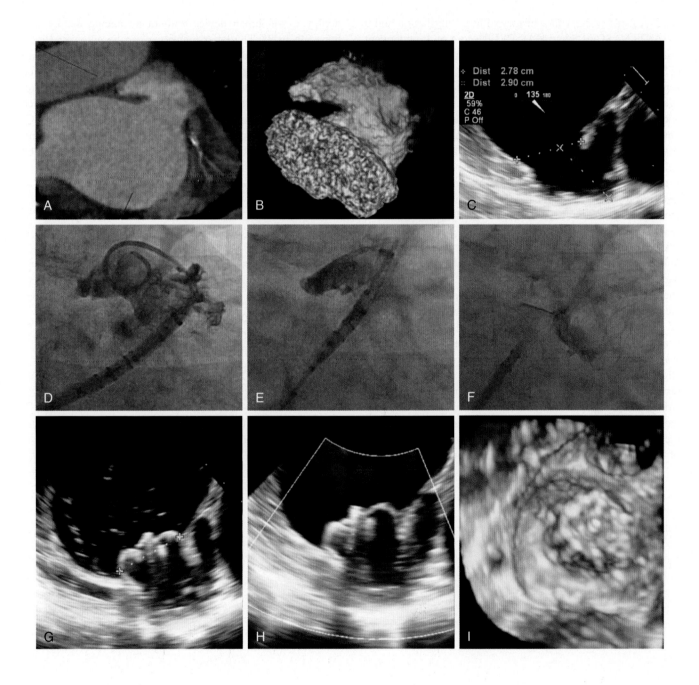

Treatment of a Chicken Wing Left Atrial Appendage

Matthew J. Price, MD

A 73-year-old man, with a history of atrial fibrillation and a CHA_2DS_2VASC of 5 and HAS-BLED score of 4, underwent left atrial appendage (LAA) closure. A transseptal puncture (TSP) within the infero-posterior portion of the interatrial septum (IAS) was performed using multiplanar transesophageal echocardiography (TEE) guidance. The LAA is an anterior and superior structure, and therefore an inferior and posterior TSP will generally provide a coaxial approach for device occlusion. A, The inferior-superior axis of the IAS is delineated by the bicaval TEE view, and the anterior-posterior axis is delineated by the basal short-axis during TSP puncture (arrow). A 6-Fr pigtail catheter was then advanced across the septum into the LAA through a double-curve Watchman delivery sheath (Boston Scientific, Natick, MA). B, LAA angiography was then performed in the right anterior oblique-caudal projection. This demonstrated that the LAA had an anterior "chicken-wing" anatomy. C, The delivery sheath was then advanced into the LAA over the pigtail catheter, but it could not be advanced sufficiently into the body of the LAA, despite aggressive counterclockwise rotation, because of the orientation of the appendage in relation to the TSP site. D, Therefore repeat TSP was performed inferior and slightly posterior to the initial site (arrow). E, LAA angiography through an anterior curve delivery sheath now demonstrated that the sheath was coaxial to the LAA, (F) allowing the sheath to be maneuvered deeply enough for delivery of the required 24-mm device. In this particular case, the neck of the chicken wing provided enough depth to successfully deploy a Watchman device without advancing deeply into the wing itself. The latter maneuver can be associated with complications, including tearing of the LAA when the sheath straightens during device advancement. Next, the device was deployed using the standard technique, and after a tug test, fluoroscopy and (H) angiography showed the device was well-positioned and (H) fully occluding the LAA. G, On TEE, the device was adequately compressed (minimum, 14%), without residual leak, and therefore released. I, The final result was confirmed by angiography.

IVC, Inferior venae cavae; SVC, superior venae cavae.

KEY POINTS

- An inferior and posterior TSP is critical for procedural success, as it provides a coaxial approach toward the LAA.
- Consider repeat TSP in an alternative location if a coaxial approach and sufficient sheath advancement into the LAA cannot be rapidly accomplished with the initial puncture site.
- While closure of chicken wing anatomy with the Watchman LAA occluder can be challenging, it can be straightforward when the LAA has sufficient depth proximal to the "elbow" of the wing.

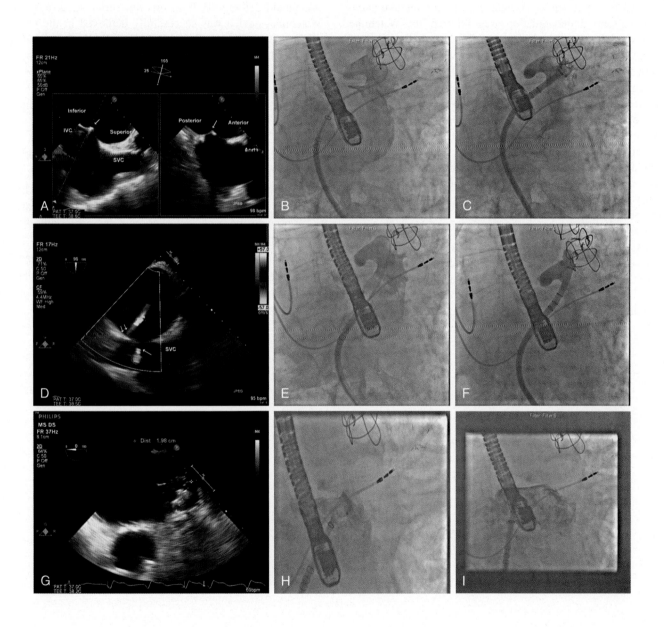

Pearls From a Case of Left Atrial Appendage Closure

Jason H. Rogers, MD, Gagan D. Singh, MD, and Thomas W. Smith, MD

An 82-year-old man with paroxysmal atrial fibrillation (CHA_2DS_2-VASc score, 5) and a need for an alternative to long-term anticoagulation was referred for Watchman (Boston Scientific, Maple Grove, MN) left atrial appendage (LAA) occlusion. Initial transesophageal echocardiography (TEE) derived measurements of the LAA were as follows: 0 degrees, 21.4 mm (ostium width) $\times$ 25.0 mm (depth); 45 degrees, 16.2 $\times$ 29.4 mm; 90 degrees, 19.2 $\times$ 27.0 mm; 135 degrees, 20.1 $\times$ 16.3 mm. A, The 135-degree view revealed a predominant posterior lobe. Therefore a single curve access sheath was selected, which orients more coaxial with posteriorly directed appendages. C, A conventional inferior and posterior transseptal puncture (TSP) was performed, and initial LAA contrast injection through a 5-Fr pigtail catheter confirmed a predominantly posterior lobe. D, The single-curve access sheath was then advanced over the pigtail into the LAA, but the access sheath was pointed superiorly, and the approach angle was not coaxial with the LAA (arrow). As a result, adequate guide depth could not be achieved. B, Therefore the TSP was repeated in a more anterior and superior location, resulting in a more favorable approach angle to the LAA. E, The single-curve sheath could then be advanced coaxial (arrow) to achieve adequate depth in the LAA for Watchman delivery. F, With this new orientation, a 27-mm Watchman device was successfully deployed in the ostium of the LAA with excellent seal and apposition. The patient was discharged home without complications, and 6-week follow-up TEE showed complete closure of the LAA.

KEY POINTS

- The default TSP location for Watchman LAA closure is inferior and posterior in the fossa ovalis.
- Although the double-curve access sheath is used in the majority of cases, the single-curve sheath can provide more coaxial alignment for posteriorly-directed left atrial appendages.
- To provide better alignment for posterior oriented lobes, a more anterior and superior location (in the mid-superior/inferior and mid-anterior/posterior fossa ovalis) is advantageous.

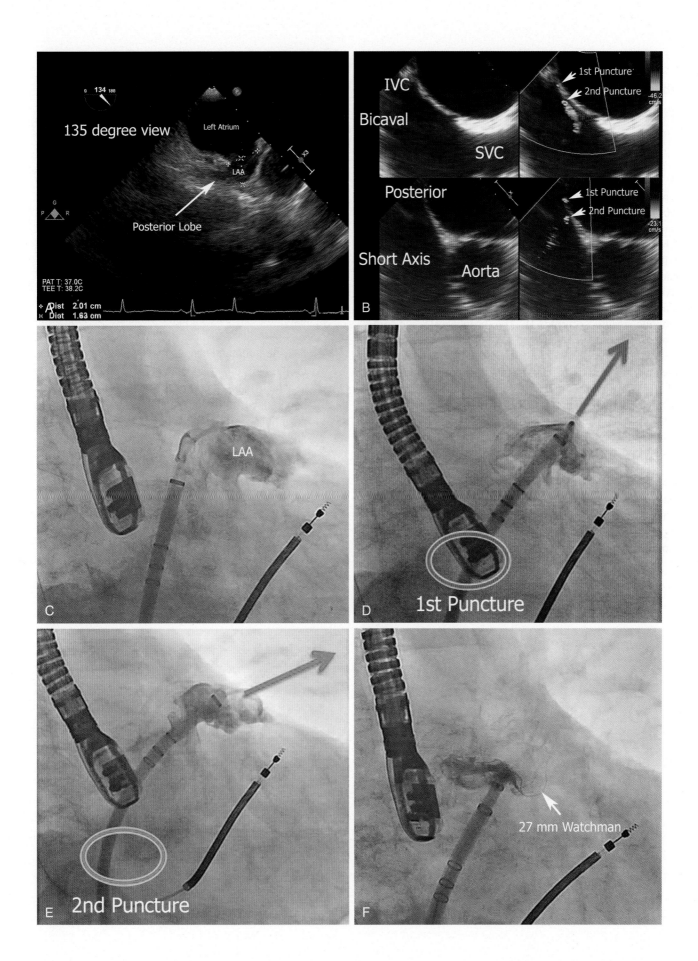

Residual Leak Treatment After Left Atrial Appendage Closure

Patrick Boehm, MD, Stefan Bertog, MD, PhD, Laura Vaskelyte, MD, Ilona Hofmann, MD, Jennifer Franke, MD, Rahul Sharma, MD, Sameer Gafoor, MD, and Horst Sievert, MD, PhD

A 74-year-old man was referred for left atrial appendage closure with a Watchman device (Boston Scientific, Natick, MA), in the setting of hypertension, atrial fibrillation, and three prior cerebrovascular events. His risk scores were CHADS2=4, CHADS2VASc= 5, and HAS-BLED=4. The left atrial appendage was a three-lobed structure, with a caudal lobe having almost a separate origin. A, The largest diameter by angiography was 22.8 mm, and a 27-mm device was implanted. At 45-day follow-up, no clinically significant embolic events occurred. B, Transesophageal echocardiogram at the 0-degree view showed a persistent leak (arrow) with ostial width of 5 mm and depth of 16 mm. Due to bleeding risk and risk of persistent stroke due to leak, closure of the leak was recommended. In the cardiac catheterization laboratory, right femoral venous access was obtained and transseptal puncture was performed under transesophageal echocardiography (TEE) guidance. C and D, The leak was cannulated with a 6-Fr multipurpose guide catheter and its severity was confirmed with angiography. E, The dimensions allowed implantation of a 10-mm Amplatzer Vascular Plug II (St. Jude Medical, St. Paul, MN) into the residual lobe. F–H, This plug effectively covered the lobe. He was treated with 3 months of daily dual antiplatelet therapy (aspirin 81 mg and clopidogrel 75 mg), followed by aspirin indefinitely.

KEY POINTS

- Residual leak after percutaneous left atrial appendage device closure occurs in almost half of patients at 45-day follow-up with TEE. For leaks >5 mm, additional anticoagulation is recommended.
- Improvement in procedural technique, device iteration, and echocardiographic visualization has led to less para-device leaks. However, leaks can potentially be thrombogenic, as they provide large access to the left atrial appendage. For those patients in which leaks are present, closure of leaks has been shown to be safe and effective. This can be accomplished through proper visualization, access, and sizing.

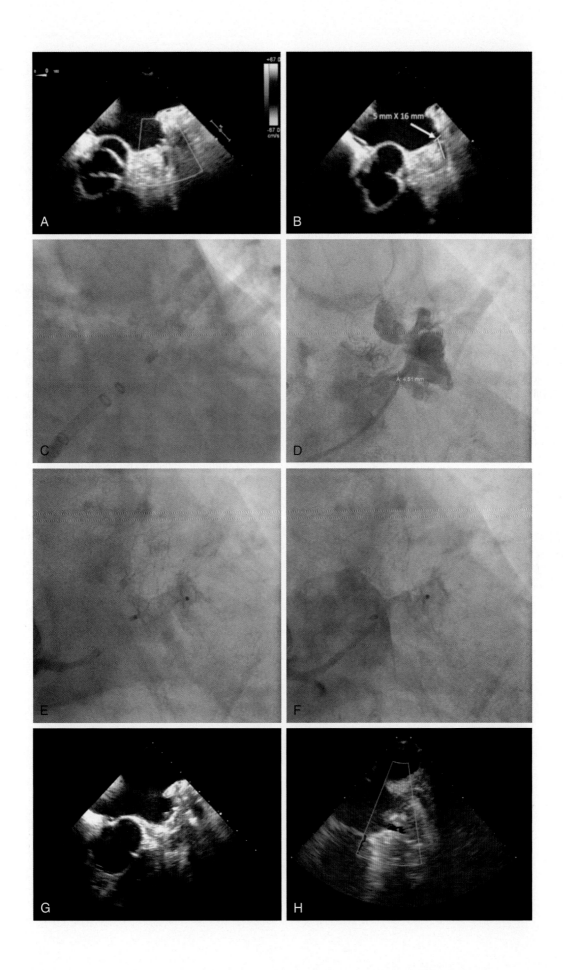

Closure of Multiple Pseudoaneurysms in the Ascending Aorta

Paul Sorajja, MD

A 54-year-old man was found to have two, large aortic pseudoaneurysms, in the setting of multiple prior sternotomies for valvular disease due to mantle chest radiation for Hodgkin's lymphoma. At his last surgery, the aortic valve was re-replaced with an 18-mm mechanical ATS prosthesis, and a root enlargement was not possible due to severe calcification. Endarterectomy was performed to remove massive calcific shelves throughout the ascending aorta and proximal aortic arch. Postoperatively, he had evidence of refractory, chronic anemia. Chest computed tomography, with axial (top) and coronal imaging (bottom), demonstrated a large pseudoaneurysm in the mediastinum that surrounded a heavily calcified aorta. A, Ascending aortography demonstrates origin of one pseudoaneurysm on the right side (arrowhead). B, A 6-Fr, Judkins right coronary guide catheter is used to engage the origin (JR), followed by passage of a 0.014″ coronary guidewire (arrowheads) and a Quick-Cross catheter (QC) (Spectranetics, Colorado Springs, CO). C, A 0.018″ Glidewire (arrowhead) (Terumo, Somerset, NJ) is inserted. D, Over the guidewire, a 6-Fr Shuttle sheath (Cook Medical, Bloomington, IN) is placed into the pseudoaneurysm. E and F, The catheter is exchanged for a 9-Fr Flexor Shuttle sheath, followed by extrusion and placement of a 38-mm Amplatzer Atrial Septal Occluder (arrowheads) (St. Jude Medical, St. Paul, MN). G, The second pseudoaneurysm is engaged and treated in similar fashion with a Judkins right coronary catheter, a 0.014″ coronary guidewire, and exchange over a glidewire for a 6-Fr shuttle sheath. H, An 8-mm, Type II

Amplatzer Vascular Plug (St. Jude Medical, St. Paul, MN) is placed (arrowhead). I, Final deployment of two devices (arrowheads). J, Final aortogram shows closure of the pseudoaneurysms.

KEY POINTS

- Aortic pseudoaneurysms can be approached with catheters and wires conventionally used to treat coronary bypass grafts. Use of soft coronary guidewires enhances steering of the coronary catheter.
- Once the pseudoaneurysm is cannulated, a step-up approach for placing stiffer guidewires is utilized with exchange catheters such as the Quick-Cross. The stiffer guide wires can then be used to place a variety of delivery catheters for deployment of device occluders.
- Complete closure is essential for pseudoaneurysm therapy, as any persistent flow will cause the pseudoaneurysm to remain patent. In this case, the first pseudoaneurysm was very large and required a 38-mm occluder for complete closure, while an 8-mm plug was sufficient for the second pseudoaneurysm.

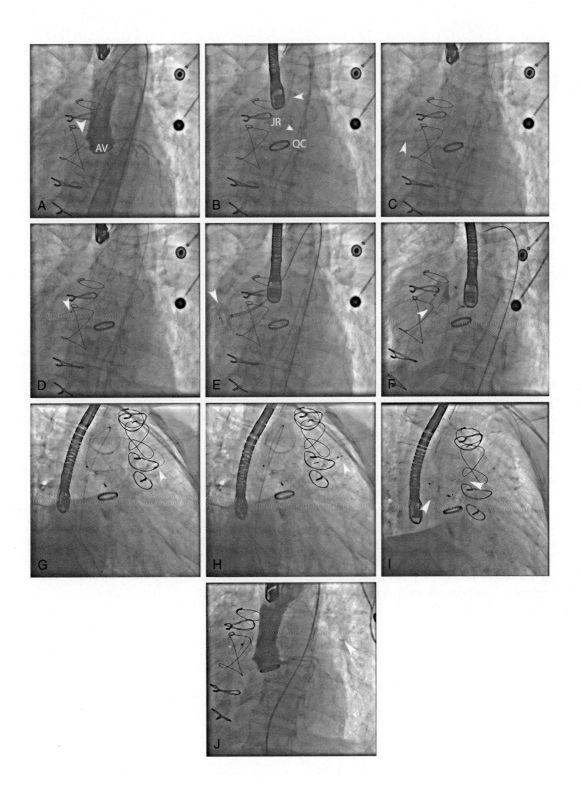

Apical Pseudoaneurysm Closure

Paul Sorajja, MD

An 86-year-old man, who was previously treated for aortic stenosis with a transcatheter self-expanding prosthesis, was found to have a large pseudoaneurysm in clinical follow-up. A and B, Transthoracic echocardiography with Doppler color-flow imaging demonstrating a large pseudoaneurysm (P) arising from the apical inferior wall of the left ventricle (LV). C, From the left chest and with echocardiographic guidance, the pseudoaneurysm is cannulated with a micropuncture needle, which is exchanged for a 0.035″, angle-tipped Glidewire (arrowhead) (Terumo, Somerset, NJ). D, The wire is passed through into the LV, aortic valve, and the descending aorta, where it is snared with a 15-mm gooseneck (arrowhead), and exteriorized through the left femoral artery. E, Through the left femoral artery, a 90-cm, 8-Fr Flexor Shuttle sheath (Cook Medical, Bloomington, IN) is advanced as a guide catheter (GC) retrograde over the rail, through the LV, and into the pseudoaneurysm. The rail is released, leaving the microcatheter in the pseudoaneurysm. The distal portion of a 12-mm Amplatzer Ventricular Septal Defect Occluder (St. Jude Medical, Fridley, MN) is then extended (arrowhead). F, The occluder is fully decoupled (arrowhead). The microcatheter is wired and removed, followed by placement of a standard 6-Fr sheath in the pseudoaneurysm. G, Through the sheath, a 12-mm type II Amplatzer Vascular Plug (St. Jude Medical, Fridley, MN) is extruded and guided into position (arrowhead) with contrast injections in the side-arm of the sheath (S). H, Final deployment of the plug (arrows) and the occluder (arrowhead). I, Intraprocedural transthoracic echocardiography showing the guide catheter (arrow) in the LV with the distal disk of the occluder (arrowhead) in the pseudoaneurysm. J, Final transthoracic echocardiogram showing positioning of the disks of the occluder on both sides of the left ventricular free wall (arrow), and absence of flow into the pseudoaneurysm on Doppler color imaging.

KEY POINTS

- Cannulation of the pseudoaneurysm directly was undertaken due to its proximity to the skin. This approach minimized the need for retrograde wire manipulation in the LV, which can be technically challenging and be associated with entanglement with the mitral chords.
- Creation of the rail enabled easy passage of the guide catheter into the pseudoaneurysm. Retrograde passage was chosen to minimize potential interaction of the distal portion of the occluder with the mitral valve apparatus.
- Access sites can be closed with vascular plugs passed through standard arterial sheaths, with guidance from contrast injections into the sheath side arm.

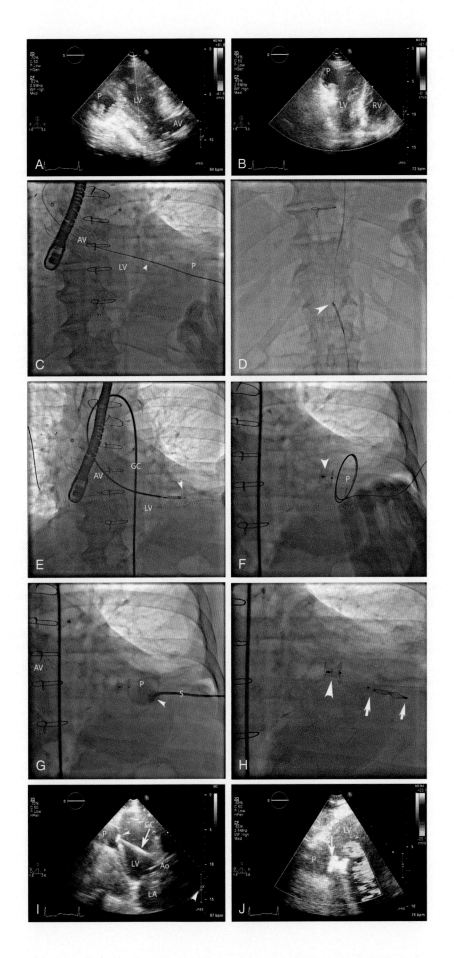

Transventricular Therapy of Pulmonary Homograft

Paul Sorajja, MD, Marko Vezmar, MD, Charles M. Baker, MD, John R. Lesser, MD, Barry Cabuay, MD, Marcus Burns, DNP, and Vibhu Kshettry, MD

A 44-year-old man presented with refractory right heart failure, in the setting of tetralogy of Fallot and multiple cardiac surgeries, including pulmonary valve homograft placement and mechanical tricuspid valve replacement (5 total prior sternotomies). The patient also suffered from Diamond-Blackfan anemia and was dependent on prednisone and periodic transfusions. The echocardiogram demonstrated severe pulmonary stenosis (gradient, 49 mm Hg) and moderately-severe pulmonary regurgitation, with marked right ventricular enlargement. After careful consideration of the options, a transcatheter approach to treating his pulmonary homograft was undertaken. Preprocedural computed tomography was performed to determine the alignment of the transcatheter with direction of the pulmonary homograft (arrows) using (A) frontal and (B) axial imaging. The right ventricle (RV) was notably shifted into the left chest. Surgical cut-down with a left thoracotomy was performed to expose the RV. Following placement of pledgeted sutures, the RV was then punctured and a 6-Fr sheath was placed. A balloon wedge catheter was used to place a standard wire, followed by a pigtail catheter. C, An aortogram was performed to ensure adequate distance from the homograft to the coronary artery. D, Baseline pulmonary angiography helps to delineate the landing zone. E, Balloon valvuloplasty with a 30-mm Z-med (B Braun, Bethelem, PA) was inflated with simultaneous aortography to help ensure coronary patency during subsequent intervention. F, A Lunderquist wire (Cook Medical, Bloomington, IN) was placed in the right pulmonary artery using a balloon wedge catheter, followed by placement of an 18-Fr Cook sheath (Cook Medical, Bloomington, IN). G, A 30-mm Palmaz-Schatz stent was hand-crimped onto a Melody BiB balloon (Medtronic Inc., Minneapolis, MN), and unsheathed across the pulmonary homograft (arrow). A 29-mm Sapien XT prosthesis (S, Edwards Lifesciences, Irvine, CA) was then advanced to the Palmaz-Schatz stent. H, Due to the coaxial nature of the access point, no flexion was required (arrowhead). The Sapien prosthesis was post-dilated with a 30-mm True balloon (Bard Peripheral Vascular, Inc., Tempe, AZ). I, The final gradient across the prosthesis (arrow) was only 13 mm Hg. Echocardiography and pulmonary angiography demonstrated no pulmonary regurgitation.

Ao, Ascending aorta; B, balloon valvuloplasty catheter; LCA, left coronary artery; PA, pulmonary artery; RA, right atrium; RCA, right coronary artery; RV, right ventricle; RVOT, right ventricular outflow tract; S, Sapien prosthesis; Sh, sheath; TV, mechanical tricuspid valve prosthesis; W, guidewire.

KEY POINTS

- For appropriate candidates (mechanical tricuspid prosthesis), transventricular placement of prostheses for pulmonary homograft therapy is possible. Careful preprocedural planning to achieve the most coaxial alignment to the pulmonary homograft helps to minimize the flexion on the delivery catheter.
- Care must be undertaken to ensure no interaction with the coronary arteries during pulmonary intervention. This potential can be ascertained with preprocedural computed tomography angiography, as well as performing simultaneous aortography during the pulmonary valvuloplasty.

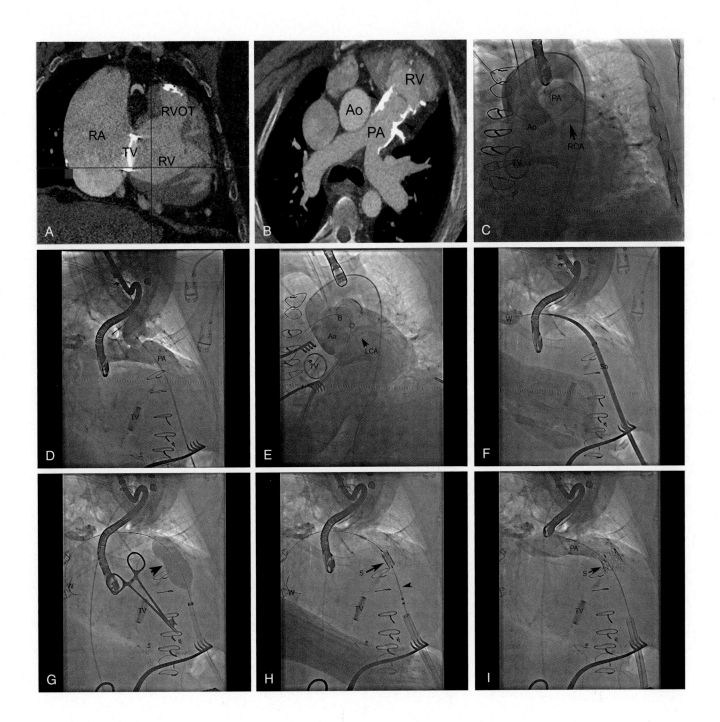

Left-to-Right Atrial Shunting Device for Management of Heart Failure With Preserved Ejection Fraction

Rami Kahwash, MD, and Scott M. Lilly, MD, PhD

A 72-year-old woman with a history of hypertension and diabetes mellitus presented with 3 years of progressive fatigue and decreased exercise capacity. Her physical exam revealed bibasilar rales and mild lower extremity edema. The echocardiogram showed preserved left ventricular ejection fraction and hemodynamics consistent with diastolic dysfunction and no significant valvular abnormalities. The brain natriuretic peptide was mildly elevated. Medical therapies were escalated, yet she remained symptomatic (New York Heart Association class III) despite optimization of volume status and adequate blood pressure control. An invasive hemodynamic study established the presence of exercise-induced elevations in pulmonary capillary wedge pressure (>25 mm Hg) with relatively stable right atrial pressure (~15 mm Hg). She was enrolled in the REDUCE –LAP HF II study, which was designed to evaluate the clinical efficacy and safety of left-to-right atrial shunting device for management of symptomatic heart failure with preserved ejection fraction. After randomization, she underwent implantation of the Intra-Atrial Shunt Device (IASD) (Corvia Medical, Tewkesbury, MA). This device was implanted in the atrial septum, with the aim of reducing left atrial pressure by permitting blood flow from the left to the right atrium. A, The device has a double-disc design that spans the atrial septum with an opening ("barrel") in the center. B–D, Using a 16-Fr sheath and a 0.035″ wire, the device (arrows) is implanted with conscious sedation from the femoral vein under fluoroscopic and intracardiac echocardiographic guidance. Her pulmonary capillary wedge pressures and the pulmonary pressures, measured (E; left = baseline, right = post-IASD) at rest and (F; left = baseline, right = post-IASD) post-exercise, were lower following implantation of the device.

LA, Left atrium.

KEY POINTS

- IASD is currently under investigation for the treatment of heart failure with preserved ejection fraction. The device creates a connection opening between the left and right atria that permits reductions in left atrial and pulmonary venous pressures, and aims to reduce exertional dyspnea.
- In select patients with evidence of exercise-induced elevation in pulmonary capillary wedge pressure, IASD may improve symptoms and functional capacity.
- Deployment of the IASD is done using a transcatheter approach via the femoral vein under fluoroscopic and intracardiac echocardiographic guidance.
- After transseptal puncture, the IASD is delivered over a 0.035″ wire, followed by exposure and retraction of the left atrial disc, then unsheathing of the right atrial disc prior to device release.

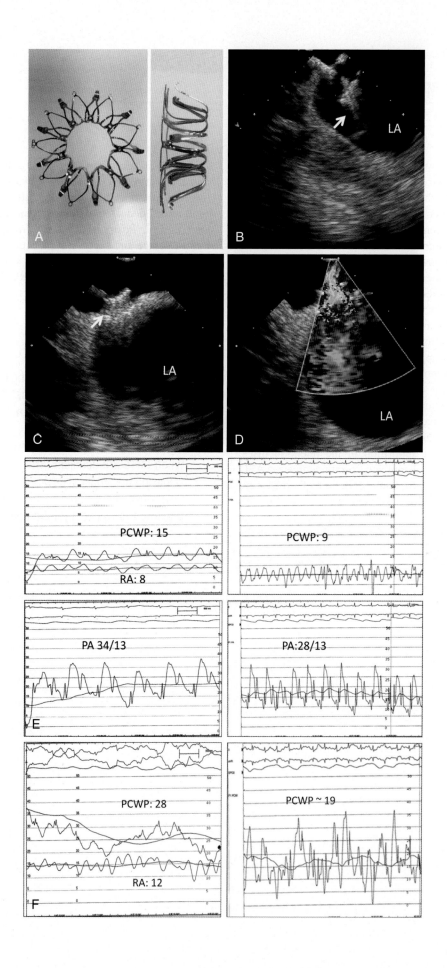

Closure of Eccentric Atrial Septal Defect

Ganesh Athappan, MD, and Paul Sorajja, MD

A 54-year-old woman with a large secundum atrial septal defect (ASD) was referred for percutaneous device closure. On echocardiography, there was a large ASD with left-to-right shunting and severe right ventricular enlargement. The defect was highly eccentric. A, On transesophageal echocardiography, the minor axis measured 18 mm (arrow). B, Adequate anterior-posterior rims were present for the defect (arrow). C, However, the inferior rim (arrowhead) was markedly deficient and was located in the majoraxis of the defect, which measured 27 mm. D, Significant shunting was present on Doppler color-flow imaging. E, Cardiac computed tomography showed the inferior rim to be 5 to 7 mm (arrowhead). Using a transfemoral approach, the ASD was crossed conventionally with a balloon wedge catheter and straight wire, followed by placement of a stiff wire and sizing balloon. Due to the eccentric nature of the ASD, sizing with a 26-mm balloon was not occlusive for shunt flow. We were concerned that the short-axis of the ASD would constrain the device occluder and not permit apposition of the retention discs. Thus we initially placed 24-mm and 26-mm Amplatzer ASO devices (St. Jude Medical, St. Paul, MN), both of which were associated with residual flow. We then were successful with a 28-mm Amplatzer ASO device. F and G, The waist of the device was constrained by the short-axis dimension of the ASD (arrowhead), raising the possibility of poor apposition. Note the relative widening of the waist of the occluder. H, However, on color-flow imaging, the retention discs were found to be adequately wide and apposed enough to occlude shunt flow. I, Postprocedural CT imaging shows the constrained device and successful placement.

Ao, Ascending aorta; AV, aortic valve; LA, left atrium; LV, left ventricle; RA, right atrium; RV, right ventricle; SVC, superior vena cava.

KEY POINTS

- Eccentric ASDs can be challenging to treat as the short-axis dimension may constrain occluders and cause the retention discs to not fully appose the atrial septum.
- These defects are therefore particularly challenging when there are deficient rims.
- Choosing the smallest device that will occlude shunt flow while maintaining stability of the occluder is important for procedural therapy of these defects.

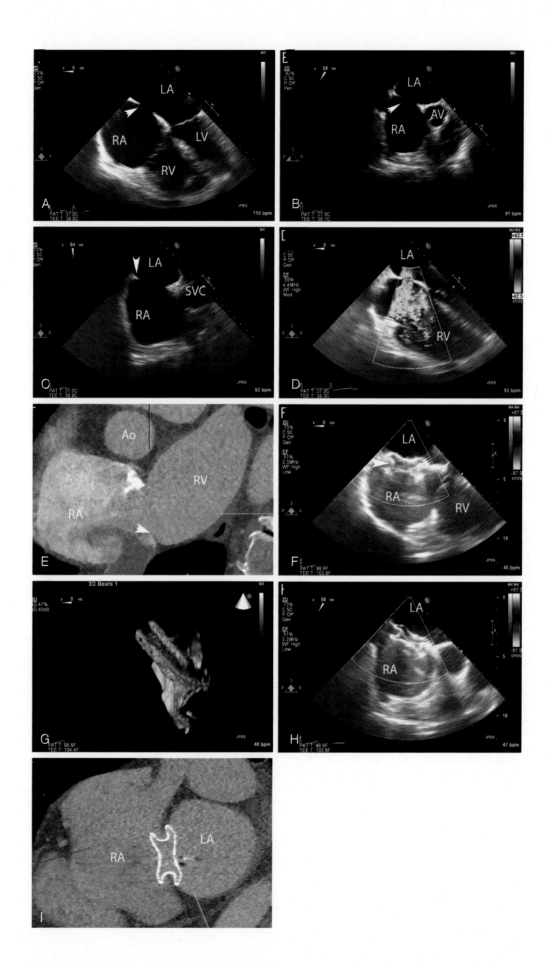

Tricuspid Disease

Transcatheter Tricuspid Valve Annuloplasty With Pledget Implantation for Severe Tricuspid Regurgitation

Ivandito Kuntjoro, MD, Gorav Ailawadi, MD, and D. Scott Lim, MD

A 65-year-old man presented with recurrent right-sided heart failure due to persistent severe tricuspid regurgitation after previous, successful transcatheter mitral valve repair with Mitraclip (Abbott Vascular, Santa Clara, CA). Transesophageal echocardiography demonstrated severe tricuspid regurgitation with (A) mild residual mitral regurgitation and (B) severly dilated tricuspid annulus. C, Using a transjugular approach, a Trialign catheter (Mitralign, Tewksbury, MA) was positioned below the tricuspid annulus to (D) deliver the wire across the tricuspid annulus. The wire tip was snared from the right atrum side. E, The delivery catheter was then inserted over the snared wire to implant the first pledget (arrow). The steps repeated to deliver the second pledget. F, Both pledgets (arrows) were subsequently plicated together with the goal of reducing the annulus size. G, Final angiogram demonstrated two pledgets with the lock (arrow) and patent right coronary artery flow. H, Diagram is shown to illustrate the final result. I and J, There was significant reduction of the annulus size resulting in improvement of tricuspid valve coaptation and reduction of tricuspid regurgitation. (I, baseline; J, post-procedure).

RA, Right atrium; RV, right ventricle; TA, tricuspid annulus.

KEY POINTS

- Transcatheter tricuspid annuloplasty with pledget implantation is a feasible alternative the treatment of functional tricuspid regurgitation.
- Multiple pledget implantations may be required to achieve optimal result.

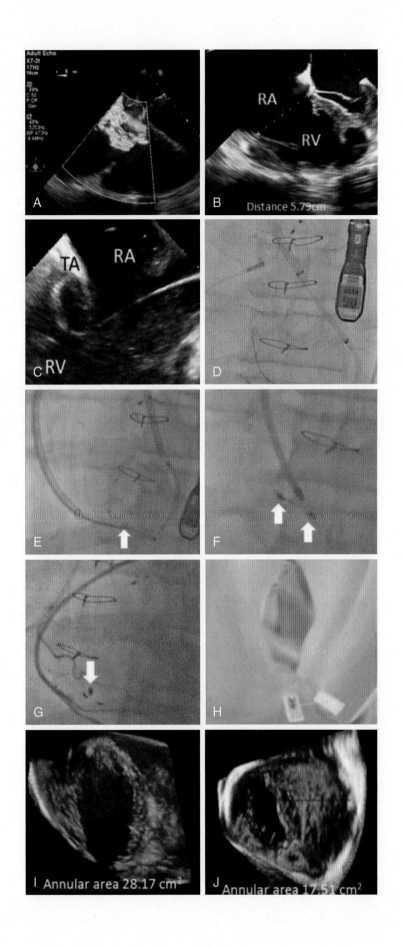

Imaging for the Tricuspid Valve: Tips and Techniques

Tanya Dutta, MD, MA, Hasan Ahmad, MD, Martin Cohen, MD, and Gilbert H. L. Tang, MD, MSc, MBA

An 85-year-old, frail woman presented with symptomatic severe mitral regurgitation (MR) and torrential tricuspid regurgitation. Her medical history included prior coronary artery bypass grafting, atrial fibrillation, hypertension, and chronic renal disease. Due to her age, frailty, and severe comorbidities, she was deemed to be an extremely high surgical risk, and underwent staged transcatheter repair. Initially, she had transcatheter mitral valve repair with placement of two MitraClips (Abbott Vascular, Santa Clara, CA), leading to a reduction in the MR from 4+ to 1+. The atrial septum was closed with an occluder. The patient remained symptomatic from her tricuspid regurgitation (arrows), which was evident on (A) mid-esophageal and (B) transgastric views. C, Adequate size of the tricuspid septal leaflet was confirmed in the 3-dimensional (3-D) imaging. A transfemoral, venous approach was used for off-label MitraClip therapy to treat the tricuspid regurgitation. D, The mid-esophageal view and corresponding X-plane image were used to confirm clip alignment (arrows). E, Leaflet grasp was performed in the same view (arrows). Clip orientation was visualized on the (F) transgastric short-axis view (arrow) with (G) guidance from fluoroscopy (arrow). H and I, A clip was deployed at the anteroseptal commissure and the tricuspid regurgitation was reduced (arrows). In follow-up, the patient had residual severe tricuspid regurgitation, but her symptoms had improved (New York Heart Association class I/II) and were medically manageable.

A, Anterior; Ao, ascending aorta; ASO, atrial septal occluder; LA, left atrium; P, posterior; RA, right atrium; RV, right ventricle; S, septal; SGC, steerable guide catheter.

KEY POINTS

- For transcatheter repair of tricuspid regurgitation, 3-D (for adequate leaflet size), transgastric (for clip orientation), and mid-esophageal (for leaflet grasp and clip deployment) views should be employed.
- Mild reductions in tricuspid regurgitation can lead to significant clinical improvement.

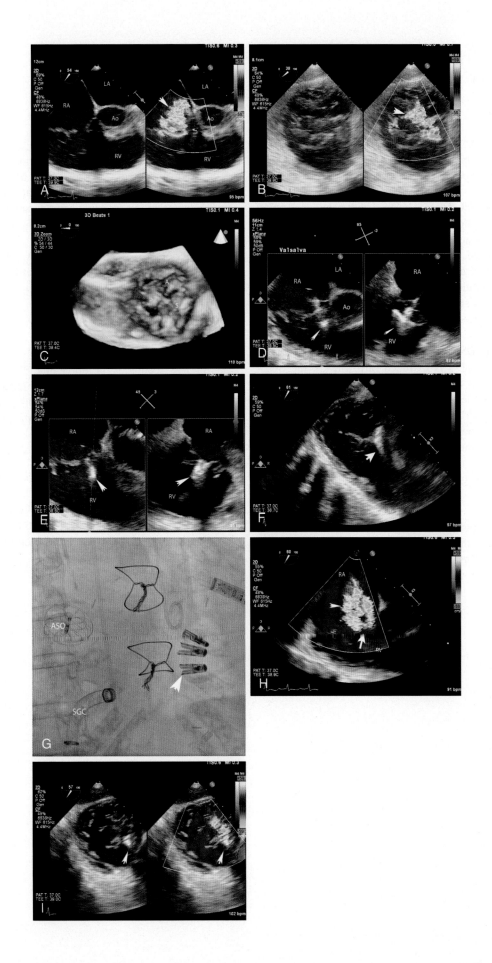

Tricuspid Transcatheter Repair

Paul Sorajja, MD

A 79-year-old woman was referred for treatment of drug-refractory symptoms of right heart failure. She had multiple morbidities, and transcatheter repair with MitraClip (Abbott Vascular, Santa Clara, CA) was undertaken. A, Transesophageal echocardiography (TEE) shows severe tricuspid regurgitation (arrowhead). B, TEE with 3-dimensional (3-D) view of the tricuspid valve from the right atrium (RA) indicates the septal (S), anterior (A), and posterior (P) leaflets. C, The steerable guide catheter (SGC) (arrow) is positioned in the RA with targeting of the posterior and septal tricuspid leaflets. This orientation is stored for reference on fluoroscopy. D, The SGC is then straightened to allow the clip delivery system (CDS) to be advanced without tension into the RA. Once the CDS is extruded (arrowhead), the SGC is then moved back to the landmarked position for crossing of the tricuspid leaflets. E, The clip (arrowhead) is then advanced across the posterior and septal leaflets (arrows) without steering from the sleeve. (F) Transthoracic echocardiography with para-apical views is used to visualize the clip arms (arrowhead) as they are retracted toward the tricuspid leaflets. G, The grippers are dropped, followed by arm closure (arrowhead). Leaflet insertion is assessed (arrowhead). H, Final echocardiographic image shows the deployed clip on the tricuspid valve (arrowhead). I, Fluoroscopic image demonstrates the position of the clip (arrowhead) prior to closing of the arms. J, Fluoroscopy shows deployed clip (arrowhead). K, TEE with 3-D imaging demonstrates the clip deployed (arrowhead) across the posterior and septal leaflets of the tricuspid valve. L, The degree of tricuspid regurgitation has been reduced to moderate (arrowhead) following clip implantation. An invasive hemodynamic assessment (M) before and (N) after clip placement shows a significant, acute drop in right atrial pressure.

A, Anterior; Ao, ascending aorta; LA, left atrium; LV, left ventricle; P, posterior; RA, right atrium; RV, right ventricle; S, septal.

KEY POINTS

- In this technique of transcatheter tricuspid valve repair with MitraClip, steering is achieved through movement of the SGC only, with employment of the plus/minus knob and through clockwise/counter-clockwise rotation.
- This approach avoids the need to "miss-key" the device, and does not require use of the steerable sleeve.
- As assessment of residual tricuspid regurgitation can be challenging, measurement of change in right atrial pressure is of incremental clinical benefit.

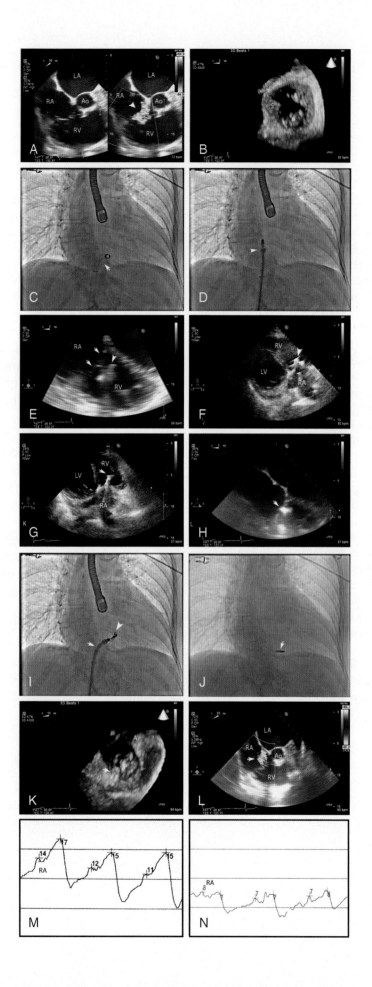

Transcatheter Tricuspid Valve Repair With the FORMA Repair System

Lluis Asmarats, MD, François Philippon, MD, and Josep Rodés-Cabau, MD

An 82-year-old woman, who had previously undergone aortic valve replacement and concomitant coronary artery bypass grafting 6 months ago, presented with aggravating dyspnea (class III). A, Transthoracic echocardiography revealed massive, functional tricuspid regurgitation due to right ventricle (RV) annular dilatation and leaflet malcoaptation. Following a heart team decision, the patient was deemed inoperable (Logistic EuroSCORE 60.7%, EuroSCORE II 18.9%) and was considered for transcatheter tricuspid valve repair with the FORMA Repair System (Edwards Lifesciences, Irvine, CA). B, Preprocedural computed tomography (CT) confirmed severe tricuspid annular dilatation (diastolic diameter 51 × 42 mm; area, 16.7 cm^2). The procedure was performed under general anesthesia, using combined fluoroscopic and transesophageal echocardiography (TEE) guidance. Following left axillary vein access, a 24-Fr introducer sheath was inserted. C, RV ventriculography (right anterior oblique, 30 degrees) was then performed to identify both the tricuspid annular plane and the target anchoring zone, located at the RV apex perpendicular to the center of the annulus. D, A steerable balloon-tipped delivery catheter was advanced within the RV and (E) the anchor was deployed at the septal portion of the RV apex. The steerable catheter was retrieved. F, The 15-mm Spacer device, a passively expanding foam-filled polymer balloon creating a platform for native leaflet coaptation, was tracked over the rail to the tricuspid annulus, aiming an ideal target device positioning of 30%/70% (right atrium and RV, respectively). Upon placement, the device was proximally locked at the subclavian region, and the remaining rail length was placed within a subcutaneous pocket. Her mean right atrial pressure decreased from 12 mm Hg at baseline to 6 mm Hg after percutaneous tricuspid valve repair. G and H, Postprocedural transthoracic echocardiography showed mild tricuspid regurgitation (II/IV). No complications occurred, and the patient was discharged 5 days after the intervention. At 2-year follow-up, her course has remained uneventful with only New York Heart Association functional class II symptoms.

KEY POINTS

- Transcatheter tricuspid repair with the FORMA Repair System may be considered for the treatment of patients with severe functional tricuspid regurgitation deemed at very high or prohibitive surgical risk.
- Careful preprocedural evaluation, including CT, transthoracic echocardiography and TEE, is crucial to assess venous access, RV anatomy, and optimal projection of coaxial anchoring site.
- Guidance of the delivery rail anchoring at the RV apex should entail both angiography (usually right anterior oblique 30 degrees) and TEE (90–120 degrees transgastric view). An additional left anterior oblique 40-degree projection might be useful to determine optimal septal orientation of the steerable catheter.
- Despite incomplete reduction in tricuspid regurgitation, early and mid-term clinical improvements in functional status, quality of life and reduction of rehospitalization are observed following the intervention.

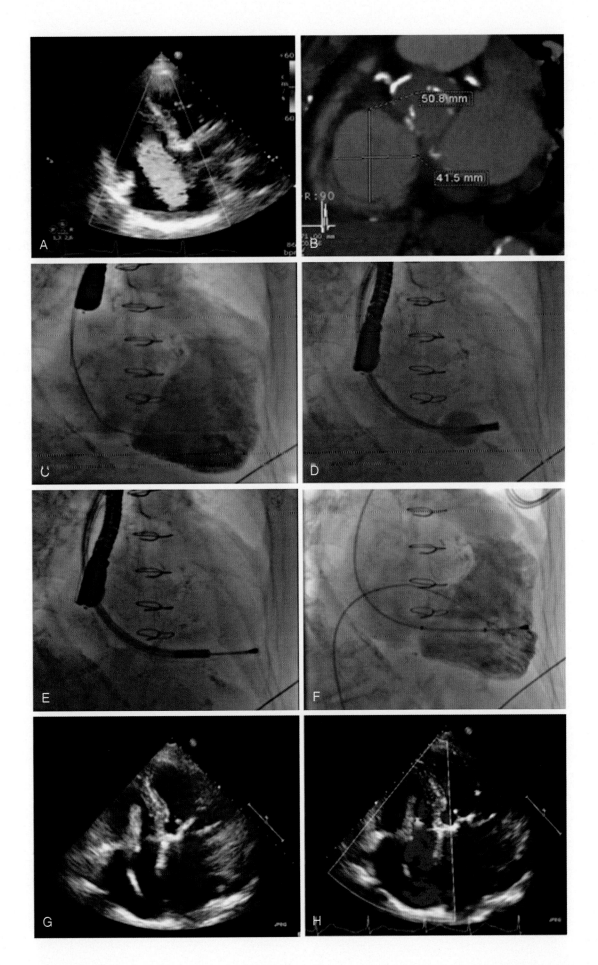

Transapical Valve in Tricuspid Ring

Evaldas Girdauskas, MD, PhD, and Eva Harmel, MD

A 57-year-old woman with progressive right heart failure and a medical history of triple valve surgery (aortic valve replacement, mitral valve re-replacement, and tricuspid annuloplasty) was admitted to hospital with acute decompensated heart failure, cardiac cachexia, and signs of multiorgan failure. Her tricuspid surgery consisted of a 32-mm Carpentier-Edwards-Classic annuloplasty ring (Edwards Lifesciences, Irvine, CA). Echocardiography demonstrated severe intrinsic tricuspid regurgitation due to leaflet tethering, with pulmonary hypertension (60 mm Hg + right atrial pressure) and reduced right ventricular systolic function (TAPSE, 10 mm). Preprocedural computed tomography revealed a ventrally located, severely dilated, and hypertrophied right ventricle with the apical segment adjacent to left parasternal chest wall. Given this anatomy, transapical access through a left anterior mini-thoracotomy was chosen for tricuspid valve-in-ring implantation.

A, A 29-mm Sapien XT prosthesis (Edwards Lifesciences, Irvine, CA) was selected for implantation. With an Amplatz SuperStiff wire (Boston Scientific, Maple Grove, MN) positioned in the superior vena cava, the Sapien prosthesis was aligned inside the annuloplasty ring. B and C, The prosthesis was deployed with an additional 2 cc of contrast saline solution under rapid ventricular pacing. Postprocedural echocardiography showed an excellent result, with mean pressure gradient of 3 mm Hg and no significant residual paravalvular or valvular regurgitation.

KEY POINTS

- Transapical approach via the right ventricular apex is a viable alternative for tricuspid valve-in-ring implantation in selected high-risk patients.
- Selection of the appropriate prosthesis size is crucial for all valve-in-ring procedures, and is chosen according to the inner ring diameter of the annuloplasty ring.

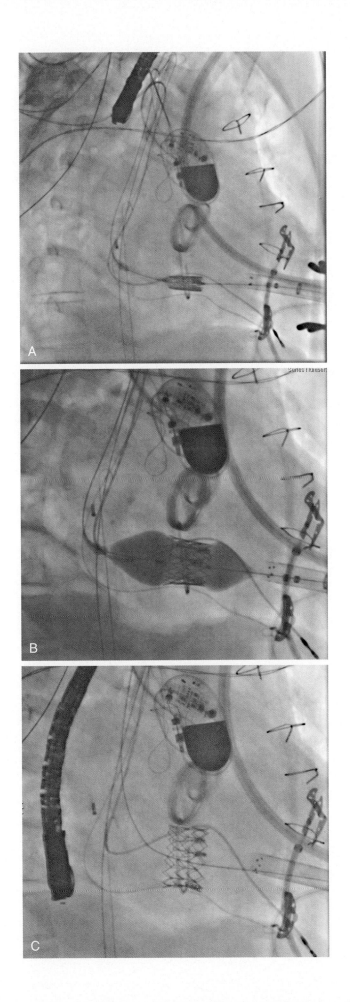

Page numbers followed by "*f*" indicate figures, and "*b*" indicate boxes.